Building Healthy Individuals, Families, and Communities

Creating Lasting Connections

PREVENTION IN PRACTICE LIBRARY

SERIES EDITOR
Thomas P. Gullotta
Child and Family Agency, New London, Connecticut

ADVISORY BOARD

George W. Albee, University of Vermont
Evvie Becker, University of Connecticut
Martin Bloom, University of Connecticut
Emory Cowen, University of Rochester
Roger Weissberg, University of Illinois
Joseph Zins, University of Cincinnati

BUILDING HEALTHY INDIVIDUALS, FAMILIES, AND COMMUNITIES:
Creating Lasting Connections
Ted N. Strader, David A. Collins, and Tim D. Noe

HIGH-RISK SEXUAL BEHAVIOR:
Interventions with Vulnerable Populations
Evvie Becker, Elizabeth Rankin, and Annette U. Rickel

REDUCING THE RISKS FOR SUBSTANCE ABUSE:
A Lifespan Approach
Raymond P. Daugherty and Carl Leukefeld

SUCCESSFUL AGING: Strategies for Healthy Living
Waldo C. Klein and Martin Bloom

SUCCESS STORIES AS HARD DATA:
An Introduction to Results Mapping
Barry M. Kibel

TYPE A BEHAVIOR: ITS DIAGNOSIS AND TREATMENT
Meyer Friedman

Building Healthy Individuals, Families, and Communities

Creating Lasting Connections

Ted N. Strader, David A. Collins, and Tim D. Noe

Council on Prevention and Education: Substances, Inc. (COPES)
Louisville, Kentucky

Kluwer Academic / Plenum Publishers
New York, Boston, Dordrecht, London, Moscow

362.2917
S8956
2000

Library of Congress Cataloging-in-Publication Data

Strader, Ted N., 1953-
   Building healthy individuals, families, and communities : creating lasting connections /
Ted N. Strader, David A. Collins, Tim D. Noe.
      p. cm. -- (Prevention in practice library)
   Includes bibliographical references and index.
   ISBN 0-306-46317-2 -- ISBN 0-306-46318-0 (pbk.)
      1. Youth--Substance use--Prevention. 2. Substance abuse--Prevention. I. Collins,
David A., 1956- II. Noe, Tim D., 1960- III. Title. IV. Series.

   HV4999.Y68 S77 2000
   362.29'17'0835--dc21

                                                                         00-023858

ISBN 0-306-46317-2 (Hardbound)
ISBN 0-306-46318-0 (Paperback)

©2000 Kluwer Academic / Plenum Publishers, New York
233 Spring Street, New York, N.Y. 10013

http://www.wkap.nl/

10 9 8 7 6 5 4 3 2 1

A C.I.P. record for this book is available from the Library of Congress

Printed in the United States of America

Preface

Youth have nearly always exhibited behaviors that frustrate adults. It can be difficult to understand why young people engage in risky or destructive behavior, and it is challenging to develop strategies to encourage more healthy and responsible behavior among our youth. However, it is helpful to realize that despite the fact that large numbers of youth engage in frightful and destructive behaviors for periods of time during adolescence and early adulthood, a large proportion of youth find a way not only to survive but also to bounce back and contribute significantly to the furtherance of human development.

We are not the first generation of adults to experience the pain, fear, and frustration of dealing with our youth. More important, we recognize that we are not helpless when faced with the problems youth experience. While it is true that adolescents have always exhibited problem behaviors, a number of effective tools and approaches have always been at our disposal to assist with appropriate youth development. Of course, the most effective approaches require a tremendous amount of focused time and energy.

Today, more than ever before, we have available to us a large body of knowledge about how to reach and influence youth, even high-risk youth and families, to help them build resiliency. This book will describe a program, Creating Lasting Family Connections, which is based on COPES's successful Creating Lasting Connections (CLC) demonstration program. CLC was demonstrated through a rigorous evaluation to have increased both family and youth resiliency. In addition, CLC showed delayed onset and reduced frequency of alcohol and other drug (AOD) use through the moderating effects of changes in youth and family resiliency factors. In this book, we will describe in detail the underlying principles that guided us in the development of this program. While our program focuses on AOD-related issues and outcomes, we believe that much of our approach will generalize to youth and families across a larger spectrum of issues and behaviors, including violence and inappropriate sexual behavior. Although none of these problems have a single cause, one common underlying issue often reported by individuals who exhibit such behaviors is their perception of isolation, abandonment, or disconnection from others. We believe our work and the general approach we have developed can assist other caring adults in influencing today's youth in positive ways, leading to impressive results.

We have found that addressing negative social behaviors like youth substance abuse, violence, inappropriate sexual behavior, and related problems is best accomplished by focusing on "influence" and "engagement" rather than control. Using influence, as opposed to control or coercion, has proved to be a very effective strategy in our efforts to affect youths' behavior. Gaining positive influence requires the development and maintenance of a meaningful relationship among the youth, families, and communities that we hope to help. Yet, surprisingly, authoritarian and overly controlling societal responses dominate our culture's attempts to influence negative or unhealthy youth behaviors. For example, at the time of the writing of this book our nation's Congress is examining legislative responses to the tragic pattern of violence in schools. The most recent occurrence, in which fourteen students and one teacher died from gunfire at Columbine High School in Colorado, has captured the attention of our lawmakers. The congressional debate involves three major approaches. Two of them are clearly attempts to control something outside of our direct relationships with youth. One is to control access to guns via age restrictions, safety locks, and other approaches; a second is to exert some control over the violent content of movies and video games. The third, which is allied to our view that it is important to make deeper connections with youth, involves the distribution of the Ten Commandments for posting in schools and classrooms across the nation. Yet the mere posting of those words on a wall is not likely to have a deep and lasting impact. At best, it would send a positive message or symbolically represent a desire to bring our youth into an appropriate social context. Unless we create programs, however, that instill a deeper sense of belonging, respect, and relationship in our most at-risk youth, our impact is likely to be minimal.

While controlling responses help adults feel good about doing something to address our nation's pain and fear, they also create a false sense of security by making us believe that we have successfully addressed the problem. At the same time, these types of controlling responses actually seem to reduce our young people's sense of connection with, and status in, the larger society. Unwittingly, we end up reducing the opportunity to develop meaningful and influential relationships with the youth we intend to impact.

Earlier we noted a pattern of negative outcomes when young people lack a sense of connectedness. These youth do not seem to be involved in meaningful ways with their larger peer groups, their families, or, most of all, their schools and communities. Parents today are clearly concerned about the safety of their children at school. They are concerned specifically about violence, gang involvement, drug use, and inappropriate sexual behaviors. They fear their children are vulnerable, both as victims of others' behavior and as subject to peer influence to participate directly in these behaviors. Our programming is designed to create deeper bonding by increasing the meaningful engagement of youth with their families, peers, schools, and the community at large. These connections are a large part of what helps prevent problem behaviors from occurring. Our programs can assist schools, churches, and other civic organizations to help parents, teachers, and others involved with youth to participate in developing strong relationships with them and implementing preventive approaches. Such approaches would include early warning systems to detect calamities like Columbine and deter them from occurring within our schools and communities. We do this by engaging our youth and their families in meaningful activities that promote a sense of connection to our larger family—the community.

By "engagement" we mean involving youth, their families, and other caring adults (entire communities) in positive ways that strengthen these relationships and develop lasting connections. A growing stream of literature underscores the importance of developing support for both individuals and families through multiple types of community engagement and support. By strengthening our young people's feelings of connection to their families and communities, we make our youth more resistant to destructive behaviors and more resilient to the long-term negative effects of destructive behaviors that occur in their lives and in our general society. A significant number of youth are growing up in our culture with very little sense of connection or social conscience. We must create a deep and lasting sense of human connection within our youth. The need to connect (and/or reconnect) our youth to themselves, their families, and their communities has never before had such a clear mandate.

PURPOSE

The purpose of this book is to describe a comprehensive, multifaceted youth substance abuse prevention program based on a demonstration program that has successfully achieved desired AOD outcomes in a variety of urban, suburban, and rural settings, and to examine the larger issue of how to promote healthy, happy, and productive youth through such programs. The Creating Lasting Family Connections program grew out of a long history of successfully engaging youth, parents, and community members in substance abuse prevention programming that works. It is our firm belief that interested communities, groups, and individuals can learn from our experience. There are, of course, many underlying principles that go into the creation of a successful prevention program. This book describes these underlying elements by using a systematic approach that explains why we have taken the approach that we have, what we have implemented in the way of programming, and what we have learned.

A larger purpose of this book, however, goes beyond a description of what has worked for us in drug abuse prevention and the people we have engaged in our substance abuse programs, and discusses how you and others can become more deeply involved in influencing and engaging today's youth in ways that are meaningful for you, our youth, and our society. For example, one of the most basic and important underlying principles we have found is to build on existing strengths, rather than attacking problems or problem people. Too often we create a negative focus and a harmful stigma for the individuals, families, and communities with whom we wish to work in dealing with a number of social problems, including drug abuse. Unfortunately, this exacerbates an already powerful sense of inadequacy, defensiveness, exclusion, and shame on the part of those needing our help. Building from strengths, rather than attacking problems, has proved to be critical to our successful program development.

Throughout this book we will examine other general principles that we have come to embrace and the specific programmatic elements we have developed that embody these principles. We hope our readers will examine our efforts and use whatever positive elements they find to develop other programs and approaches that are helpful and effective.

We have a wealth of experience in developing, implementing, and evaluating programs that are successful,* yet we clearly understand that neither we nor anyone else can write the universal program. Each of us must bring our own talents and strengths into the approach we personally choose to implement. In a very real sense, effective prevention is conducted by people who feel a deep sense of personal ownership in their efforts and connectedness with those they wish to influence in positive ways.

---

*Creating Lasting Family Connections (CLFC) was developed from our original Creating Lasting Connections (CLC) program, which was a 5-year high-risk youth demonstration project funded by the Center for Substance Abuse Prevention. Throughout this book, when we discuss outcome evaluation results, these refer to the original research on CLC (in Johnson, et al., 1996).

Acknowledgments

This book could not have been accomplished without the assistance and support of many people. The impetus for this book grew out of an evaluation conducted on our Creating Lasting Connections (CLC) program. While COPES had created these curriculum materials privately, the evaluation was conducted under a Center for Substance Abuse Prevention (CSAP) High Risk Youth Grant (SPO 1279). We have many to thank at CSAP including the director, Dr. Karol Kumpfer, and within CSAP's Division of Knowledge Development and Evaluation the director, Dr. Paul Brounstein, and the acting deputy director, Dr. Stephen E. Gardner. Special thanks go to Tommie Johnson Waters, formerly of CSAP, and now director of the Division of Prevention Services, Arkansas Bureau of Alcohol and Drug Abuse Prevention. We also must acknowledge Dr. Knowlton Johnson of Community Systems Research Division of the Pacific Institute for Research and Evaluation, who was the principal investigator in our original CLC program evaluation. Dr. Michael Berbaum, research scientist in the Institute for Social Science Research at the University of Alabama, is acknowledged for his significant contribution to the data analysis. Ms. Linda Young, president of the Community Systems Research Institute, Inc., also made a significant contribution to the development of the evaluation tool kit for the Creating Lasting Family Connections (CLFC) program. A debt of gratitude goes to our editor at Kluwer Academic/Plenum Publishers, Tom Gullotta, for his encouragement and careful review of many drafts of the manuscript. We gratefully acknowledge the help of Father Joe Merkt for his planning, conceptualization, and vision in the CLC program development. We appreciate Barbara Stewart and Mike Townsend of the Kentucky Division of Substance Abuse who have provided continuing support to COPES over the years. Special thanks are also due to George and June Merrifield and the St. Jude Foundation for their generous donations of time and resources. In addition, we would like to thank both current and former staff members at COPES for their help and support on this and many other projects: Kim Roberts, Warrenetta Crawford Mann, Vickey Strader, Carolyn Overall, Jackie Alexander, Chris Hunter, Stan Hankins, and Esther Frederick. We would also like to acknowledge the contribution of a number of people who influenced the development of the CLFC curriculum: Lena DiChicco and Dr. Ruth Davis, developers of the CASPAR Education Program, Alcohol and Drug Curriculum Series, Dr. George Mann of St. Mary's Hospital in Minneapolis, Jim Crowley of Community Interventions in Minneapolis, Stephen Glenn's Developing Capable People program, and the National Institute of Drug Abuse's training programs, including Drugs in Perspective. Finally, we would like to thank all of the youth, parents, teachers, and other caring individuals who have allowed us the opportunity to share our programs with them and their families over the years. We've learned much of what we share in this book from those with whom we have had the privilege and honor to work.

About COPES

The Council on Prevention and Education: Substances, or COPES, Inc., is a private nonprofit organization dedicated to providing youth, families, and other caring adults with effective programs designed to promote the healthy development of youth and to enrich family living.

COPES originated through an innovative project operated by the Roosevelt Community School Board of Louisville, Kentucky, in 1976. In 1981, COPES was formed as a separate private nonprofit drug abuse prevention service organization. Since its inception, COPES has provided primary prevention consultation and training to the faculty and staff of over 200 schools. In addition, consultation and training have been provided to more than 250 local agencies and organizations and more than 10,000 individuals.

In 1989, COPES was awarded a 5-year $1 million federal demonstration grant (grant number SPO #1279) from the Office of Substance Abuse Prevention (now the Center for Substance Abuse Prevention) for the Creating Lasting Connections (CLC) program. CLC was designed as an ecumenical, community-based program that focused on increasing community, family, and individual (youth) protective factors that would lead to delaying the onset and reducing the frequency of alcohol and other drug use among at-risk 12- to 14-year-olds. In 1995, COPES received a $1.1 million grant to adapt the CLC program for implementation in a number of local youth recreational centers.

COPES programs have received numerous awards for excellence. In 1988, COPES received a Federal Letter of Commendation from the Secretary of Health and Human Services, Otis T. Bowen, M.D. In 1989, the COPES Prevention Program was recognized as one of 20 Exemplary Prevention Programs by the Office of Substance Abuse Prevention. COPES's CLC project also received the Center for Substance Abuse Prevention's Exemplary Prevention Program Award for 1995.

In 1995, CLC was included in the International Youth Foundation's YouthNet International, a directory of the most effective youth programs in the world. Finally, CLC was one of only seven model prevention programs selected by the Center for Substance Abuse Prevention for national dissemination in 1998.

Contents

The Need for Prevention

*Efforts to control alcohol use and related problems . . .
can be traced back over 3,600 years to the oldest written
code of law, the Code of Hammurabi, which contained
regulations regarding the sale of alcoholic beverages
(Moskowitz, 1989, p. 54).*

Before providing an analysis of our program, it is helpful to view a "snapshot" of current trends in youths' alcohol and other drug use, and to review several historical approaches to prevention in the United States. It is important to understand the extent, nature, and historical context of any social problems we are trying to alleviate through policies and programs. Thus, we will briefly track the history of policies and approaches already attempted. In doing so, we will see that many of the approaches used to address problems such as youth substance abuse prevention have been misguided, uninformed, and largely unsuccessful.

First, let's examine the current dimensions of the youth substance abuse problem in the United States at the dawn of the twenty-first century. Then we'll look back at some of the major types of preventive efforts implemented over this century to get a view through the "rearview mirror."

The 1998 Monitoring the Future study indicated that 52% of U.S. 12th graders in the poll had used alcohol in the previous 30 days; for 10th graders, the use rate was 39%, and for 8th-graders, 23% (Johnston, O'Malley, & Bachman, 1999). Of greater concern, however, are the figures on heavy drinking by youth. The same Monitoring the Future report showed that nationally 31% of 12th graders polled reported having five or more drinks in a row within the previous 2 weeks. For 10th graders, that rate was 24%, and for 8th graders, 14%. We know that many public health and social problems result from under-age abuse of alcohol. These problems range from injuries and deaths caused by car crashes to school dropouts, delinquency, and alcohol-related aggression and violence.

In addition to other risks associated with youth alcohol consumption, Wagenaar (1993) reports that young drinkers are at higher risk for later addiction to, or problems with, alcohol. Preventing patterns of regular drinking may therefore have benefits even beyond adolescence and into adulthood.

Marijuana is the third most often used substance of abuse among youth (following alcohol and tobacco). The figures for previous-month use of marijuana were 23% of 12th graders, 19% of 10th graders, and 10% of 8th graders (Johnston et al., 1999). In addition, small yet significant percentages of students reported use of cocaine and inhalants. For example, 4.8% of 8th graders reported previous-month use of inhalants, and 2.4% of 12th graders reported previous-month use of cocaine.

For both youth and adults, alcohol and other drug (AOD) abuse issues are intimately tied to other societal problems. For example, youth violence, including gang violence, is a growing concern in our society. Kingery, Pruitt, and Hurley (1992) found evidence in a representative sample of U.S. adolescents that drug users, compared with nonusers, were involved in more fights and also were more likely to be victims of assaults. Clearly, a set of complex relationships exists between substance use and violence, but regardless of the nature of the relationship, aggression and substance abuse are plainly linked. Pransky (1991) demonstrated that many social behavior problems (among them alcohol/drug abuse, delinquency, and teen suicide) have many contributing factors in common. In addition, interconnecting relationships have also been found between the various problem behaviors themselves. In a recent analysis by Greenblatt (1998), youth aged 12 to 17 who reported using marijuana in the past year (in a national survey) also reported a variety of problem behaviors—and the greatest difference between users and nonusers was in delinquent behavior (including use of alcohol or drugs for nonmedical purposes, cutting classes, and stealing). The author points out that while conclusions about causality cannot be reached from these statistics, there is a strong positive correlation between self-reports of problem behaviors and self-reports of marijuana use. More broadly, drug use in general is strongly correlated with virtually every other problem behavior demonstrated by young people. The list of correlates includes the full spectrum of violent and antisocial behaviors. Pransky (1991, p. 31) links the problem of AOD abuse with 10 other social problems, which include teen suicide, delinquency (including violent behavior), domestic violence, and AIDS/sexually transmitted diseases. As stated earlier, a central and pervasive sense of isolation, exclusion, and/or disconnection exists among individuals who engage in a persistent pattern of behaviors seen as inappropriate by the larger society.

EBB AND FLOW OF RESPONSES

The previous snapshot of the current alcohol and drug situation in the United States indicates a clear need for substance abuse prevention. Let's look at that snapshot as one frame of a moving picture. Just as there are constant fluctuations in the levels of use of certain drugs (e.g., cocaine use by 12th-grade students), there are also rises and falls in drug use in general. We want to emphasize that the ebb and flow in the trends of alcohol and drug usage in our history has been marked by a concomitant ebb and flow in societal and governmental reactions to the prevailing patterns of drug use in our society. U.S. history reveals cyclical rises and falls both in social drug use and in societal responses of prevention, legislation, and/or eradication. In his book *The American Disease*, Dr. David Musto (1987) chronicled the rise and fall of both drug use and our nation's attempts to respond to the cyclical increases in use with preventive measures. He argued that societies typically pass through three stages related to drug usage. First, there is a stage of euphoria, as a small group experiments with the substances. In this stage, specific "new" drugs are discovered that bring relief or pleasure, and there are few reports of negative effects. Second, there is a middle period in which usage expands to a wider group and more negative effects begin to emerge. Finally, there is a period of rejection as the general popular image of the substance becomes negative. This three-stage cycle can be seen in the history of opiates, cocaine, LSD, marijuana, and many other substances.

Interestingly, our nation's ability to respond is often so slow that by the time we recognize that a problem exists and become emotionally charged enough to engage in a focused "preventive" effort, the use of that substance has usually already begun to decline, often as a result of a collective experience of negative consequences. For example, Musto points out that one cycle of drug use in the United States began between 1965 and 1970 when a significant percentage of the population began to use drugs of various types. By the early 1980s, a growing backlash against alcohol abuse and illegal drug use was evident, but this backlash occurred only after many Americans had already begun to quit smoking, reduce consumption of alcohol, lose interest in the drug scene in general, and pay better attention to their health.

Musto (1987) points out that as a society we often revisit and, regrettably, recycle historic attitudes toward drugs. For example, he cited a prominent drug expert as saying in 1974 that "Cocaine . . . is probably the most benign of illicit drugs currently in widespread use. At least as strong a case could be made for legalizing it as for legalizing marijuana. Short acting—about 15 minutes—not physically addicting, and acutely pleasurable, cocaine has found increasing favor at all socioeconomic levels in the last year" (Musto, 1987, p. 265). This view was reminiscent of the 1880s, when cocaine had first appeared commercially and when it was viewed as a harmless cure for many ailments (p. 7).

Musto adds that just as during the prior wave of cocaine use (from the 1880s to World War I), the perception of cocaine changed radically from that of an apparently harmless tonic to "that of a fearful substance whose seductiveness in its early stages of ingestion only heightens the necessity of denouncing it" (p. 274). By the mid-1980s, the public furor over cocaine use had reached its highest point; again, many of the common images of cocaine as a drug mirrored those common in the first decade of this century (p. 274).

Musto's example suggests the need for developing an ongoing preventive effort that provides consistent and clear messages about drugs on a regular basis since the public seemingly has such a short memory regarding the harm substance abuse causes. We know that the snapshot of substance use we presented earlier will change and that the moving picture of substance use will reveal new trends. Some new drug or new method of administration will replace another in the current picture. But what isn't likely to change regarding drugs is the big picture. The big picture in the United States is likely to continue to involve some form of the old standards: alcohol, tobacco, and marijuana, and more important, some levels of substance use, abuse, and dependency. We would argue for a more reasoned, consistent, ongoing, and pervasive effort throughout society regardless of the current trends. This effort would include a core area of activity that connects and/or reconnects those youth among our population who feel disenfranchised, ignored, unaccepted, or excluded as a means of addressing the correlated negative behaviors that include violence, inappropriate sexual behavior, and other problem behaviors.

A SELECTED REVIEW OF HISTORICAL TRENDS IN SUBSTANCE ABUSE TREATMENT AND PREVENTION

At this point, a brief review of historical trends in substance abuse prevention will demonstrate that attempts to address drug abuse problems have taken many forms over the years.

Distinguishing between Treatment and Prevention

Interestingly, throughout much of U.S. history, we have failed to recognize that treating drug addicts is very different from providing preventive programs to general populations. In the United States, efforts to provide treatment for addicts are often confused or comingled with efforts to provide prevention for the uninitiated. This creates confusion and frustration on both fronts. As Helen Nowlis (1975) pointed out, it is important to make at least gross distinctions between the various types of drug use, such as experimental use, casual or occasional use, regular use, and heavy or compulsive use. Nowlis likewise points out that it is also crucial to distinguish between different types of users. While this is a complex matter, "acceptance of such complexity enables one to begin to define a particular problem in a community and to begin to solve it" (Nowlis, 1975, p. 16).

In our prevention programs, including CLFC, we make a clear distinction between use, abuse, and chemical dependency (or in the case of alcohol, we make a distinction between drinking, becoming drunk, and becoming alcoholic). Understanding these differences is an important first step in distinguishing between the needs of different *subgroups* within a targeted population.

Drug Replacement

Let's look at a variety of U.S. "drug prevention" efforts and the irony of how they played out over time. One often-repeated approach to problems of chemical dependency has been to replace one drug addiction with another addiction. Smith (1975) points out that when morphine was first separated from opium and began to be used in the United States in the early 1800s, physicians thought that the new opium derivative was nonaddicting and hoped it would cure opium addiction in patients. As a result, the drug was prescribed often. Levine (1974) noted much the same trend with heroin. After heroin was first produced commercially in 1898, the general opinion was that the drug was the ultimate cure for morphine and opium addiction, and physicians used the drug to treat a variety of ailments. As we all know, heroin abuse became a problem that persists to the present time.

Other examples of drug replacement have included the use of methadone to treat heroin addiction after the Vietnam war and the use of cocaine to treat morphine addiction. Drug responses to drug problems are often only minimally effective in treating current drug addicts. With heroin, for example, a treatment tool became the next big treatment and prevention problem.

Law Enforcement as Prevention

One early approach to prevention focused on legislation and enforcement as a primary method. Before the turn of the twentieth century, morphine, heroin, and cocaine were sold in this country as remedies, and an estimated 250,000 Americans became addicts. The Harrison Narcotics Act of 1914 made a number of drugs illegal under federal law (Casey, 1979). This act was a direct reaction, and a zealous one, to the growing problem of addiction to opiates. It defined addicts as criminals and assumed prevention would occur for the uninitiated simply through legislation.

Alcohol prohibition efforts in the United States culminated in the passage of the Eighteenth, or "Prohibition," Amendment. Between 1920 and 1933, the manufacture, sale, and consumption of alcohol were prohibited, but ultimately this legal remedy failed. Casey (1979) pointed out that, as with other substances, legislation "failed to create a general climate of abstention. And where there was a populace of willing consumers, supply was still able to keep pace with demand" (p. 97). While some positive effects also resulted from Prohibition, the results were widely mixed at best.

In an important work, Helen Nowlis (1975) succinctly described the "moral–legal" approach to prevention. She noted that this model was based on punishment and the threat of punishment for drug possession and use. The obvious assumption is that punishment and the threat of punishment will deter undesired behaviors. This also assumes that addicts can quit on demand, and that making a popular drug illegal will result in an immediate end to its popularity and use. Again, this approach combines and confuses treatment and prevention motives.

Another characteristic of the "moral–legal" approach is that it creates an "us" versus "them" mentality for the people and drugs that are targeted. In the history of prohibition of certain substances, drugs have often been associated with particular minority groups. For example, in the 1930s, marijuana use was often connected with Latinos. As W. L. White (1979) points out, "it is doubtful that any of the legislators in 1937 could have even conceived of the possibility of large numbers of their own grandchildren and great grandchildren using marijuana and going to jail under a legal precedent they set" (p. 174). The punishment model, even when it does not stigmatize certain minority groups, still has an impact on those who use substances, as Dennis Jaffee (1974) pointed out. Jaffee noted that young drug users often seem to view laws against drug use as part of the "context against which young people struggle to define themselves and grow" (p. 329). The young tend to be rebellious, and laws become part of the total "system" they rebel against. Further, making drugs illegal and creating harsh penalties often drives up the cost of these drugs. High drug prices create an attractive economic incentive for becoming involved in the sale and distribution of those drugs that are currently in demand. This creates a vicious cycle of incentives and disincentives that feeds a number of problematic outcomes.

Fear as Prevention

The use of scare tactics is another prevention approach used in the United States. Beck (1998) describes the history of drug policy and control under Harry Anslinger, who was commissioner of the Federal Bureau of Narcotics (FBN) (now the Drug Enforcement Administration) from 1930 to 1962. Through Anslinger's efforts, media campaigns were launched that included headlines such as "The New Narcotic Menace." Many documented "the horrible crimes committed by marijuana-intoxicated youth." Beck notes that the efforts of the FBN in the 1930s could be described as the first federally sponsored drug education campaign, and these efforts were characterized by the use of scare tactics and sensationalism and the repression of scientific information (Beck, 1998). One result of such campaigns designed to scare both addicts and the general public is that members of both groups become cynical and distrustful, and lose connection with the government or others who deliver the campaigns, which means they have low success with both groups.

The social disengagement of young substance abusers may actually increase the number of dysfunctional behaviors in which they engage. A good illustration is provided in Elaine Casey's (1979) description of federal efforts to control heroin in the 1960s. She noted that despite increased prevention efforts, heroin use continued to rise. One factor Casey cited for this is that young people had heard too many warnings that they knew were exaggerated or simply false. The young drug users "believed that government and medical indictments against the substances came from ignorance, fear, and hostility toward the youth culture" (p. 119). Casey also noted that people in the 1960s were familiar with different drugs, having tried them and used them occasionally (or even regularly). Their experience in using the substances made the exaggerated claims of the scare tactics more obvious. The resulting situation may have made it even more difficult for people to understand the real, though less obvious, problems that evolve subtly with continued substance experimentation, long-term use, and potential dependency.

"Information Only" as Prevention

A third prevention effort can be called the "information only" approach. The optimistic view of those who promote an informational approach is that giving people enough information will result in reduced use and abuse for abusers and complete avoidance by others. Again, this assumes that addicts can and will quit because they know a drug is harmful. Most addicts already know firsthand the risks involved but feel helplessly trapped anyway. And for the uninitiated, it is clear that accurate information is only a small part of what it takes to help youth or adults to make responsible decisions.

Michael Goodstadt (1986), in an article on school-based drug education efforts in the United States, noted that one failure of drug educators has been a lack of understanding concerning the building blocks of all programs: first, changes in knowledge; then in attitudes; and ultimately in behavior. Goodstadt observed that knowledge can be impacted by different programs, with varying degrees of effectiveness. However, "improvements in knowledge are a necessary, but not sufficient, condition for most behavior change" (Goodstadt, 1986, p. 278).

EXAMINING THE IMPACT OF OUR MOTIVATIONS ON PREVENTION PRACTICES

It is important to realize what the previously cited approaches (such as information-only, replacement of addiction with other addictions, and punitive approaches) say not only about how we address the problems of substance use and abuse but also what they say about us. Our motivations and feelings impact our approaches. What roles do our emotions and our judgments play in our prevention efforts?

Given what we know about the seriousness of problems associated with alcohol and drug abuse, it is common to see similar responses in parents and other caring adults—responses that emerge out of fear, anger, ignorance, or confusion. Our experience has shown that such feelings need to be recognized, named, and shared by those concerned for and trying to assist others in avoiding substance-related problems. Unless these feelings are addressed, and unless some level of comfort is achieved with the difference between treatment for addicts and prevention strategies for others, "prevention" efforts will continue to be met with resistance or avoidance on the part of youth, and frustration or burnout on the part of prevention workers.

Finally, let's look at how each of us may be motivated to engage in prevention and how our own personal motives may impact our approach and our results. To illustrate how one's own emotions may hinder efforts toward prevention, consider the following example. Let's say we are motivated primarily out of love for our children and fear of drugs. We logically might resort to helping our children fear the drugs too. Yet to scare someone enough to keep them from using a substance would require focusing on the very negative effects of a long-term pattern of heavy drug use. Such an approach would ignore the fact that it is possible for some to use alcohol and other drugs in lesser quantities and frequencies without experiencing extremely negative consequences. Young people may rightly conclude that such one-sided messages are exaggerations or distortions, and as a consequence may doubt the credibility of those who use such "scare tactics." Framing discussions in terms of potential risks versus potential benefits is much more effective, yet preventionists often find this approach somewhat uncomfortable.

In a similar way, the emotions of hurt and anger can shape prevention efforts. Feelings of anger often engender action toward a specific target. If the problem being addressed is alcohol or drug abuse, action motivated by anger might take the form of targeting the availability of a substance and the people who use and distribute it. Although prohibition, enforcement, and punishment may result in arrests and confiscations, they may not result in reduced demand for the substance. Again, as with the scare tactic approach, the punishment approach may cause a loss of connection or relationship between the youth and the adults who are trying to prevent problems. This is not to say that availability should be ignored as a factor in substance use/abuse. Rather, it suggests that we must keep in sight the individual, his or her motivation to use or abuse a given substance, and the individual's meaning to us as a society.

In addition to feeling fear and anger, a sense of frustration, helplessness, and isolation is also common as we attempt to engage in prevention efforts. It is not uncommon for us as a society at times to drop into a blind trance of defeat or to adopt a pervasive (but unrecognized) denial of substance abuse-related issues.

Ultimately, those who understand and accept the frailty of the human condition and know the power we each have to love, nurture, and support each other toward increased strength and resilience are motivated out of a sense of personal and social responsibility to make the world a better place. These individuals are somehow able both to take life as it is and yet work to improve the human experience as they encounter others in their personal and professional lives. This type of motivation often engenders a calmness and patience that leads to the long-term ability to make a positive difference for themselves and others over time.

PREVENTION THEORY TODAY

At the start of this chapter we acknowledged that youth have always exhibited behaviors that scare, challenge, and frustrate caring adults. We also looked at how adults, and society in general, have attempted to shape more healthy behaviors in youth, particularly in relation to substance abuse. We saw that sometimes the means that adults and the larger society use to try to generate changes in youth are counterproductive. In this chapter and the next, however, we explore some more recent approaches to prevention that are based on theoretical models and empirical evidence. We will also show how our own program model was developed.

In many ways, we are better off than our counterparts in prevention were just a few decades ago. Bonnie Benard (1991) pointed out that during the 1980s prevention experts increased their reliance on community-based prevention, as opposed to focusing solely on the classroom and the school domain. This shift in emphasis was in line with theories suggesting that young people face pressures that may lead to problem behavior from sources outside the school setting. Johnson and Solis (1983) pointed out a number of limitations in solely school-based prevention programs, including the fact that the majority of most young people's time is spent outside of school and that both the family and the wider community outside the school have important influences—both positive and negative. According to Johnson and Solis, the optimal prevention program would use not only school systems but also families and communities. Further, such programs would be "comprehensive and highly integrated, with each component contributing according to its unique potential" (Johnson & Solis, 1983, p. 78).

Our own experience in the field of prevention affirms these community-based theories. COPES's experience has been that prevention programs focusing solely on the school domain are less effective than broader approaches. This is so at least partly because they often fail to involve parents and other caring adults in the larger community—adults who play such an important role in the lives of youth.

There is a growing recognition of prevention efforts that are based on the results of empirical research regarding both the causes of substance abuse and the effectiveness of prevention programs (Center for Substance Abuse Prevention, 1997; National Institute on Drug Abuse, 1997a). Risk and protective factors now form a part of the conceptual frameworks for many of today's prevention programs. Understanding the specific risk factors related to substance abuse in a target population is important. Program developers need to select strategies and approaches that have the greatest potential for addressing the specific risk and protective factors that are most changeable in the target population. Protective factors have also been the subject of considerable research in recent years. Emily Werner (1989) found that a significant percentage of children exposed to negative risk factors in their environments nevertheless exhibited adaptive and positive behaviors. Protective or resiliency factors are a little more complex than risk factors, and continued research on the role of protective factors in substance use and abuse by adolescents is needed.

COPES has been successful in implementing community and family-based prevention programs that integrate the use of current theories of causality in substance abuse and in participating in rigorous evaluations to show what works in our programs and why it is working. The external evaluation of CLC was extremely rigorous in that it used random assignment of youth and families to either a program group or a control group.

While it is very difficult to hold together a multiyear demonstration project that involves youth, their families, and community advocate teams, it is extremely important for prevention professionals to be able to do so. Our field has a strong need to demonstrate scientifically valid results. This book describes the CLFC model in terms of how it was designed and is being implemented. We will explain how we accomplished positive results for youth, families, and communities through the CLC demonstration project from which CLFC was developed. As others compare our efforts with their own, we hope they will discover new ways to improve the potency of their efforts and improve their results as well. In this way, we hope to add to the understanding and knowledge within the field of prevention. Our ultimate hope is to see a more clear and consistent national strategy evolve in the field of prevention.

A successful broad national strategy will require many people in many roles across many communities working together to encourage the selection of the more healthy options available to our youth. Preventionists cannot be expected to do the whole job. Actually, we do very little by ourselves. We know, through experience, that we can be successful only through positive "influence" and broad "engagement." Both of these terms suggest the humility with which we approach the difficult problems described in this chapter.

In Chapter 2, we review resiliency theory, which provided us with a theoretical basis for the development of the CLFC program. Readers who are not interested in the scientific and theoretical aspects of our specific program design might wish to move directly to Chapter 3 for a more concrete description of our programming that resulted from the science.

What Works Today in Prevention

RISK AND RESILIENCY THEORY

It is doubtful that research will ever be able to fully explain why some youth engage in alcohol, tobacco, and other drug use and others do not. It has, however, identified a number of conditions that correlate with the use of alcohol, tobacco, and other drugs among children and youth. These correlates, or risk factors, can be grouped into six major life areas or "domains"—the individual, family, school, peer group, neighborhood/community, and society/media. Each domain represents an important sphere of influence in the lives of children and youth. This view of correlates by life domains has evolved from ecological theory and is visually represented in Figure 2.1. Although our research was conducted on substance abuse prevention, it is known that virtually all other problem behaviors share many (if not most) of these same risk factors.

The relationship of these domains to a young person is frequently represented as a series of concentric circles with the youth in the center. These concentric circles depict the close to the more distant influences, so that the second circle represents the family, the third the school, and so forth, with the last and largest circle representing society. Thus, the model includes persons, events, experiences, and establishments not only in the youth's immediate environment but also in the youth's broad social milieu, including such influences as the media, advertising, and major sociocultural institutions. While society/media appears distant from the individual, there is much evidence that factors in the larger society and the media play a role in youth substance use. For example, Saffer (1991) in a study using data from 17 countries found that alcohol advertising bans had significant positive effects in reducing alcohol abuse. In another study related to the influ-

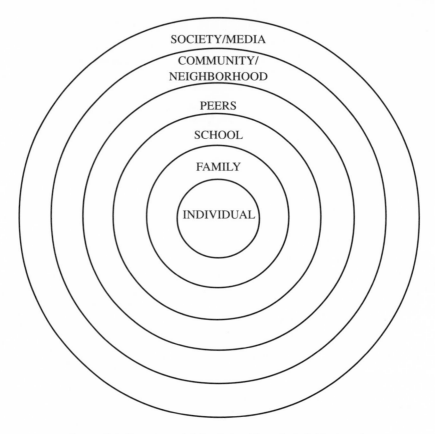

Figure 2.1. Domains and their relationship to the individual youth.

ence of advertising, Atkin, Hocking, and Block (1984) found that among adolescents who reported higher levels of drinking there appeared to be higher exposure to "lifestyle" ads promoting alcohol consumption.

The precise nature of the links between alcohol, tobacco, and other drug use and all of the individual risk factors that can be identified in the six domains is not fully understood. The research simply suggests that youth who experience risk factors in multiple domains are at increased risk for using alcohol, tobacco, and other drugs. We know also that youth who experience these risk factors in multiple domains are at increased risk for a large number of other destructive behaviors, including violence and delinquency. Many believe that prevention programs that intervene to reduce risk factors in several of these important spheres in children's lives have a greater probability of success than programs with a more limited focus. Johnson and Solis (1983), using results from a well-known heart disease prevention program, argued for using family, school, mass media, and community organization components in substance abuse prevention programs.

Our own programs and research offer additional evidence that multiple interventions in multiple domains are more effective than narrow approaches.

Recent research has identified a large number of risk factors for each of the six domains. These risk factors can be divided into two categories. The first category includes contextual issues. These are broad societal and cultural factors that provide the legal and normative expectations for behavior. The second category entails factors that lie within individuals and their interpersonal environments (Hawkins, Catalano, & Miller, 1992).

In each of the domains, conditions and experiences that appear to protect youth from initiating alcohol, tobacco, and other drug (ATOD) use can also be identified. Since some risk factors for ATOD use may be difficult to change, research into resiliency factors has become increasingly important. In other words, the impact of unchangeable risk factors may be moderated by protective (or resiliency) factors (Garmezy, 1985; Werner & Smith, 1982). Research has shown that many youth appear to moderate these negative effects and successfully resist persistent exposure to risk factors, even when there are multiple and severe risks (Werner & Smith, 1982).

The relationship between resiliency and risk factors, however, is often not obvious, because resiliency factors are not merely the reverse of risk factors. For example, Brook, Brook, Gordon, Whiteman, and Cohen (1990) reported that parent conventionality and strong attachment between parent and adolescent reduced the risk presented to youth of associating with drug-using peers. What this example illustrates is that the relationship between parents and youth (a resiliency factor in the family domain) can offset risks associated with drug-using friends (a risk factor in the peer group domain). Clearly, the risk and resiliency factors in the example are not simple opposites. This example underscores that the search for resiliency factors is not necessarily restricted to a simple reversal of a known risk factor.

Brook et al. (1990) identified two mechanisms through which resiliency factors reduce risk for youth drug use. The first is a *risk/resiliency* mechanism through which a known exposure to risk for ATOD use is moderated by the presence of resiliency factors. For example, the positive bonding relationship between a parent and youth can moderate the negative exposure of the young person to drug-using peers. The second is a *resiliency/resiliency* mechanism through which one resiliency factor enhances another resiliency factor, strengthening its effect. For example, a strong bond between a father and child can enhance the effects of other resiliency factors such as adolescent conventionality.

APPLYING THE THEORY—BUILDING FROM STRENGTHS

In designing a prevention program, practitioners must make several decisions in regard to program design. First, they must decide within which domains they can realistically stimulate corrective actions. Second, they must decide which risks and/or resiliency factors to target within the chosen domains. In designing the CLC research project and, later, the CLFC program, we devoted our energies to designing a multiple component prevention strategy. This approach targeted resiliency factors in three of the six domains: (1) community, (2) family, and (3) individual youth (Johnson et al., 1996). In the later version, CLFC, the school domain was added with the intent of building on existing strengths within even more domains.

We adopted a *resiliency/resiliency* mechanism for the original CLC program design, and this is continued in our CLFC program design. As stated earlier, through this mechanism, preventionists seek to increase resiliency factors, which may enhance other resiliency factors, strengthening the overall effects. Thus, our approach seeks to build on strengths instead of working to reduce the deficits (risk factors). We believed that some risk factors for ATOD use are very difficult to change. For example, it is very difficult to alter the low socioeconomic status of a community or even a family, a major risk factor for substance abuse. Therefore, we focused on enhancing the conditions and experiences that appear to protect youth from initiating ATOD use (resiliency or protective factors) regardless of low socioeconomic status. Our experience and past research had shown that resilient youth can avoid drug use and abuse, even when multiple and severe risk factors are present. Further, enhancing strengths is also perceived as a more positive event for individuals, families, and communities. The likelihood of stigmatization is dramatically reduced when programs focus on strengths.

The community domain's influence on ATOD use among youth has long been recognized in terms of resiliency factors that influence youth (Benard, 1991). Moreover, the recognition of relationships between community-level factors and ATOD use has caused an increased effort among preventionists to gain a broader level of community involvement in substance abuse prevention activities (Hawkins et al., 1992; Kaftarian & Hansen, 1994). Central to these community initiatives is empowerment, whereby people and groups gain mastery over their affairs (Bandura, 1986; Florin & Wandersman, 1990; Rappaport, 1987). In Chapter 3, we will point out the resiliency factors, including empowerment, targeted by the community mobilization component of CLFC.

Within the family domain, a number of resiliency factors have been viewed as important. Of particular relevance were parental knowledge and beliefs related to AOD use (Barnes & Welte, 1986; Kandel, Simcha-Fagan, & Davies, 1986); effective family management, communication, and interaction (Reilly, 1979; Tec, 1974); appropriate parental modeling of alcohol use (Barnes, 1990; Brook, Whiteman, Gordon, & Brook, 1988; Hansen et al., 1987); and appropriate family involvement in help-seeking in the community (Werner & Smith, 1982). The family domain appears to influence youth risk of AOD abuse in a number of ways. Hawkins and colleagues' (1992) key work on risk and protective factors for adolescent substance abuse problems listed the following as important factors. Family modeling of drug use and parental attitudes toward children's drug use have been shown to be correlated with AOD abuse, while poor parenting practices, high levels of family conflict, and low bonding between parents and children seem to increase the risk for a large variety of adolescent problems, including AOD abuse (Hawkins et al. 1992, p. 82).

First, looking at modeling of drug use within the family, Ahmed, Bush, Davidson, and Iannotti (1984) found evidence that "salience," which indicated the number of household users of a drug and the degree of a youth's involvement in parental drug-taking behavior, best predicted both expectations to use and actual alcohol use. Salience was also important in predicting children's cigarette and marijuana use. Therefore, increasing the likelihood of appropriate modeling of drug use through our program should help create a protective environment.

Research has also shown that parental substance use *alone* cannot explain how parental system factors relate to adolescent substance use (Anderson & Henry, 1994). Other parental behaviors, including poor and inconsistent family management practices, appear to increase the risk of adolescent drug abuse. For this reason, developing positive family management practices early on should create a more protective environment.

Hawkins et al. (1992) cite at least four types of poor and inconsistent family management practices: unclear expectations for behavior; poor monitoring of behavior; few and inconsistent rewards for positive behavior; and severe and inconsistent punishment for unwanted behavior (p. 83). In an often-cited study, Reilly (1979) found that families of adolescent drug abusers were characterized by negative communication, inconsistent and unclear behavioral limits, and unrealistic parental expectations for their children. Also in the family domain, high degrees of family conflict and low levels of bonding are correlated with a number of problems, including adolescent drug abuse (Hawkins et al., 1992). In the area of conflict, for example, Simcha-Fagan, Gersten, and Langner (1986) found use of heroin and other illegal drugs strongly associated with parents' marital discord. Interestingly, it appears that the extent of parental conflict is associated with negative behavioral outcomes among children, even in samples where all homes are broken (Hawkins et al., 1992, p. 83). Our program focuses on increasing bonding and appropriate family management skills, which should lead to reductions in family conflict.

In terms of bonding within the family, a number of researchers report a correlation between lack of parent–child closeness and initiation of drug use (Brook, Lukoff, & Whiteman, 1980; Kandel, Kessler, & Margulies, 1978). The converse has also been demonstrated – positive family relationships appear to discourage initiation (Hawkins et al., 1992). Clearly, the family plays a key role in the risk of substance use and abuse. In a recent article, Dishion, Kavanaugh, and Kiesner (1998, p. 208) noted that there is a growing consensus among intervention researchers that parenting practices are "at the center of the causal process."

Later, as we describe the CLFC conceptual model, the reader will see how attention was given to family resiliency factors that address many of the correlates noted in the literature. In addition, the focus on resiliency within our program helped us avoid stigmatizing or blaming either the youth or their parents.

Individual resiliency factors are also important correlates of adolescent substance use and abuse. Key factors that have been found to be important in prevention programming are knowledge and beliefs about AOD use (Kandel et al., 1986); life skills, including communication, social and refusal skills (Gurian & Formanek, 1983; Volk, Edwards, Lewis, & Sprenkle, 1989); and individual involvement in help-seeking (Werner & Smith, 1982).

Hawkins et al. (1992) also describe a number of individual-level risk and protective factors that are correlated with youth substance use and abuse. Included are attitudes and values favorable to drug use. A number of researchers have found that initiation into use of any substance is preceded by values favorable to its use (Kandel et al., 1978; Krosnick & Judd, 1982). Low degrees of bonding to parents and bonding to school are also related to adolescent drug use (Hawkins et al., 1992, p. 93). In terms of protective factors, Hawkins et al. (1992) delineate four elements of bonding that have been shown to be inversely related to drug use: strong attachment to parents, commitment to school, regular involvement in church activities, and belief in the "generalized expectations, norms, and values of society" (p. 96).

Life skills, including communication, social and refusal skills, are recognized as important protective factors in the individual (youth) domain. The National Institute on Drug Abuse lists as one of its key prevention principles for children and adolescents that programs should include skills to resist drugs when offered, strengthen personal commitments against drug use, and increase social competency (including communications, peer relationships, self-efficacy, and assertiveness) (National Institute on Drug Abuse, 1997b). CLFC incorporates both general social skill training and drug-specific skill development.

Help-seeking is another individual domain resiliency factor. Feldman, Stiffman, and Jung (1987) found a positive relationship between the amount of help received by families from formal and informal sources and children's behavior in school.

CONNECTEDNESS

A key factor that we believe transcends each of these domains is "connectedness." In the individual domain, connectedness means being able to recognize and name one's own thoughts and feelings. In the family domain, connectedness means feeling connected to one's family and significant others, along with being able to express personal thoughts and feelings with them. In the community domain, connectedness means discovering that one's self and family is rooted in and connected to others, including the broader community, in ways that are significant and meaningful. In the school domain, connectedness includes commitment to school and a feeling that one is comfortable in that environment and connected to one's peers. Feeling or perceiving one's self to be connected across several domains appears to create a protective shield, an immunity and a resiliency to negative influences. We have found that it is through these connections that individuals, families, and communities build resiliency and the strength to resist problem behaviors. For us, connectedness is a critical protective and healing force in human beings—young or old, rich or poor, male or female. Deep, healthy human connections build strong protective shields to prevent harm and to provide both nurturing and healing support, even when misfortune penetrates this shield.

As we stated in the introduction, youth who engage in problem behaviors commonly express feelings of isolation and estrangement. Most of us recognize that there is a sometimes seductive draw to engaging in unhealthy personal and social behaviors. These negative behaviors tend to appear gratifying in the immediate moment, while becoming broadly destructive in the long run. We believe that by assisting youth to develop a greater sense of connection with their own thoughts and feelings and a greater sense of connection with others, they develop a greater degree of immunity or resistance to these somewhat attractive yet destructive behaviors. Deeper connections appear to lead to greater immunity. Therefore, we sometimes describe our program as one that assists youth, families, and communities to foster "connect-immunity."

3

A Prevention Program that Works
Creating Lasting Family Connections

In Chapter 2, we began explaining the "why" of our approach to youth substance abuse prevention. We pointed out that research has shown relationships between young people's access to a variety of resiliency factors in a number of domains and their susceptibility to substance abuse. We also noted that a key step in developing a scientific prevention program is to identify the specific domains in which it will be implemented and the resiliency factors it is expected to affect.

In Chapter 3, we turn to the "what" of CLFC. That is, we describe the actual makeup of our program. In doing so, however, it is important to relate the "what" to the "why." Without a clear linkage between what is being implemented and why it is being implemented, prevention programs run the risk either of showing no effects or of not being able to explain why any effects that are shown might have occurred.

THE CLFC PROGRAM MODEL

The main program components in CLFC consist of community mobilization, school mobilization, parent and youth trainings, and early intervention and follow-up activities. The sections below summarize each of the main program components in turn. Following this brief summary of each component, we will present our conceptual model that pulls all of the parts together and illustrates how each contributes to a successful prevention program.

Community Mobilization

The CLFC program begins with community mobilization. Our experience, and the research on our programs, has shown that this component (which addresses the community domain in a direct way) is critical to successful program implementation. Often program developers overlook this domain and begin their program descriptions assuming that the community has already been sufficiently mobilized and has the infrastructure required to successfully implement preventive interventions. For us, this ignores the important role of the local community. This section provides a brief overview of how we mobilize and empower communities through the development of Community Advocate Teams. Later, in Chapter 5, we will examine our community mobilization strategy in greater detail.

The community mobilization component of the CLFC program is designed to positively affect community engagement as determined by the Community Advocate Teams' (1) success in recruiting families for the CLC program, (2) empowerment to participate in the program and evaluation implementation, and (3) ongoing support for community-based ATOD prevention programming.

In our work, we have identified five key stages of development for effective community mobilization. Stage I is the selection and recruitment of sponsoring organizations; Stage II is the recruitment and development (i.e., training) of the community advocate team; Stage III is the advocate team's actual recruitment of families from the community to participate in the CLFC training modules, evaluation, and follow-up; Stage IV involves advocate team participation in retention activities designed to maintain ongoing participation of families from the community (which is extremely important in such community-based prevention programs); and Stage V is community capacity enhancement. In Stage V, the community demonstrates increased responsibility, capacity, and long-term commitment for ongoing prevention programming (i.e., program continuation). A complete description of the CLFC community mobilization model is provided in Chapter 5 for readers interested in a more detailed understanding of this program component.*

School Mobilization

If the community implementing CLFC is a school community, or if a school or a number of schools play an important part in the implementation effort, then a central component of the program is school mobilization. This component, which has been added to the original CLC program model to provide additional enhancement of youth and family resiliency, was not evaluated in the original CLC research.

---

*Johnson, Noe, Collins, Strader, and Bucholtz (in press) also present the underlying theory of the community mobilization component.

The targeted outcomes at the school level in such an implementation are empowerment, participation in project activities, and improved school climate.

The local school plays an enormous role in a young person's perception of the community. The mobilization of schools in the implementation of community-coordinated prevention activity for youth and families dramatically increases the potency of resiliency-building efforts across multiple domains. When the community, school, church, and family all promote and support a clear position on an issue such as substance abuse, the negative influences elsewhere become much less attractive.

Parent and Youth Trainings

The next program component is the parent and youth trainings. These trainings are the more familiar building blocks or components of prevention programs. Our parent and youth trainings were designed to increase parent resiliency by improving parents' (1) knowledge and beliefs regarding ATOD abuse, (2) family management skills (i.e., expectations and consequences for both positive and negative youth behaviors), (3) communication skills, (4) family role modeling of alcohol use, (5) involvement in community activities with their youth, and (6) use of community services, including alcohol and other drug treatment services if needed.

The CLFC youth trainings were designed to increase the resiliency of youth by positively affecting their (1) "Getting Real" communication and refusal skills,[†] (2) bonding with their family, (3) self-reported involvement with their parents in community activities, and (4) use of community services when personal or family problems arise, especially problems related to a family member's alcohol and/or other drug use.

Early Intervention and Case Management Services

In developing the CLFC program, we realized that another key component of fostering resiliency in families would be an ongoing support system for family members engaged in the program. Therefore, early intervention, which includes problem assessment and development of a treatment/referral plan, is another component of the program model.

Follow-up case management services are also part of the program model. In CLC (the research model), case management services consisted of bimonthly telephone consultations and/or personal home visits with referral service to participants needing additional outside support. Generally, a case manager provided these

---

[†]"Getting Real" communication refers to a specific type of communication that will be described more fully later in this chapter under training components.

services for about 6 months following completion of the parent and youth trainings outlined below.

THE CLFC CONCEPTUAL MODEL

The brief sections above described the four main program components of CLFC—community mobilization, school mobilization, parent and youth trainings, and early intervention and case management. Figure 3.1 below shows the "conceptual model" for CLC.[‡] This model illustrates the program in a way that links program components and expected outcomes. While a conceptual model may appear complex at first, we have found that using the conceptual model helps keep program staff, evaluators, and interested community members focused on the targeted behavioral results. The reader can see that each of the protective or resiliency factors mentioned in the sections above is included in the conceptual model.

The reader will also note the arrows in Figure 3.1. These illustrate the types of effects hypothesized in the evaluation of our CLC program (Johnson et al., 1996). The figure has been modified to fit CLFC through the addition of the school mobilization component.

The solid lines in Figure 3.1 denote "direct effects." For example, it is expected that the CLFC program components (shown in Box 1 of Figure 3.1) will directly impact the protective factors within the community, school, family, and individual (youth) domains. This is shown in the solid lines connecting Box 1 with Boxes 2 through 5.

The dotted lines denote "moderating effects," in which, for example, positive program effects in youth resiliency (Box 5) are enhanced by positive changes in parent resiliency (Box 4). This is shown by the dotted line from Box 4 down to the solid line connecting Box 1 (program components) to Box 5. The reader is referred to Johnson et al. (1996) for complete details on the evaluation of CLC.

In addition to the conceptual model shown on page 23, another tool that outlines the CLFC program components and their anticipated immediate and long-term effects is the CLFC logic model. The logic model is described fully in Appendix B.

DETAILS OF CLFC PARENT AND YOUTH TRAINING COMPONENTS

The section above outlined the main CLFC components and showed (through the conceptual model) how the various components are expected to contribute to outcomes. This section describes the specific CLFC parent and youth trainings in

[‡]The conceptual model for CLFC was developed from the conceptual model for CLC, the CSAP demonstration project for high-risk youth and their families. The CLC conceptual model appeared in Johnson et al. (1996).

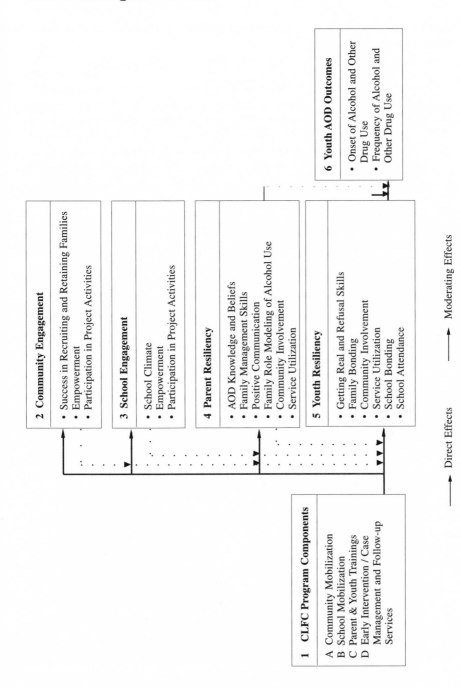

Figure 3.1. Conceptual model for CLFC.

detail. As a starting point, Figure 3.2 illustrates the specific youth and parent trainings provided in the CLFC program.

In the youth trainings, Developing a Positive Response is designed to help youth build a foundation for making appropriate decisions about AOD use. Later youth trainings build on this foundation. The Developing a Positive Response training helps youth become aware of their deepest wishes for their own health regarding alcohol, tobacco, and drugs, their relationships with others, and their yearning for success. The next youth training, Developing Independence and Responsibility, focuses on youths' current level of responsibility within their family life, with an eye toward developing personal responsibility and independence for adulthood. This training exposes young people to the potential responsibility and independence they will have in the future. It is designed to motivate them to develop the skills necessary to succeed. It also helps young people to become more sensitive to the responsibilities their own parents currently face. The Getting Real Communications Training for youth teaches the participants to understand the various types of communication styles, to recognize their own styles of communication, and to establish new patterns of interaction with family members and peers that incorporate the skills of self-awareness and mutual respect.

For parents, there are also three separate trainings. The first training, Developing Positive Parental Influences, is provided separate from, but simultaneously with, the youth training, Developing a Positive Response. In Developing Positive Parental Influences, parents and other caring adults are trained to effectively influence youth regarding alcohol and drug issues through greater awareness of facts and feelings about drugs, as well as a greater understanding of intervention, referral procedures, and treatment options. The next training for parents, Raising

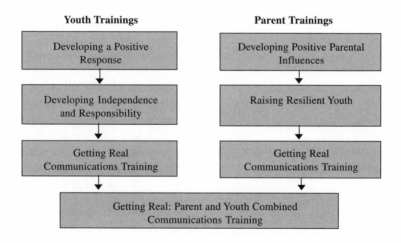

Figure 3.2. CLFC youth and parent trainings.

Resilient Youth, is designed to enhance parents' abilities to develop and implement expectations and consequences for their children in all areas of concern, including AOD use. The goal of this training is to help parents see the value of having their children participate in the setting of expectations and consequences. This encourages dialogue and bonding between parent and child. The third parent training module is the Getting Real Communications Training, which parallels the youth Getting Real training. Finally, as shown in the diagram, parents and youth come together in a combined parent and youth Getting Real training. This is an important component because it allows the youth and adults to come together to both demonstrate and practice the skills they have already learned among their own peers.

The main printed sources of information about the CLFC youth and parent training modules are the training manuals developed by COPES (1998a–e).

Full Training Module Descriptions

Each of the parent training modules ordinarily lasts about 5 or 6 weeks, with a single weekly 2½-hour session. Each of the youth training modules also lasts about 5 or 6 weeks, with a single 1½-hour session per week. The optional parent and youth combined Getting Real communications training usually requires an additional two or three meetings (with each meeting lasting 2 to 2½ hours). We have found the trainings to be most effective when parents and youth are engaged in all six training modules consecutively and simultaneously. The trainers may present the modules in any order desired, but when implementing the modules with both parents and youth participants, it is important to pair the matching parent and youth modules.

Underlying Premises of the Trainings

In the introduction, we said that we would not only describe *what* we did in CLFC but also explain the importance of certain underlying principles. Before turning to the details of each training component in our program, we provide some of the basic premises of the entire CLFC program as follows (brief lists of premises that are especially important for each specific training component are given later in this chapter):

1. No one can control someone else's behavior 24 hours a day, 7 days a week, for 18 to 21 years.
2. We can influence children through open and honest communication, including listening, sharing, and modeling. We can also share knowledge, information, understanding, and love.
3. Independence and responsibility are learned through practice.

4. Extreme attitudes and behaviors can be dangerous because children tend to adopt either the extreme position held by the parent or sometimes the opposite extreme position, leading to both internal and external conflict.
5. Pain is a natural part of life. It is normal to feel pain.
6. When a person hurts, it helps him or her to express feelings and believe that someone has listened and understood these feelings.
7. It is one thing to drink, another thing to get drunk, and something altogether different to be alcoholic or chemically dependent.
8. It can be considered neutral (neither right nor wrong) for an American adult to choose to drink a single serving of an alcoholic beverage.
9. It can be considered irresponsible to get drunk or intoxicated.
10. Anyone who consumes alcoholic beverages is at some risk for becoming an alcoholic.
11. Anyone who consumes mood-altering drugs is at some risk for becoming chemically dependent.
12. Alcoholism and chemical dependency are treatable and help is available.
13. Everyone deserves to feel accepted and included in their family.
14. Every family deserves to feel accepted and included in their community.

These premises underlie each of the different trainings described in this chapter. In the descriptions of each separate training component, other premises that are specific to that component alone will also be listed.

Developing Positive Parental Influences

This is a highly interactive alcohol and other drug issues training designed for parents and other caring adults interested in influencing youth in positive ways. Participants are expected (1) to increase their awareness of both facts and feelings about chemical use, abuse, and dependency; (2) to review effective approaches to prevention; and (3) to develop a practical understanding of intervention, referral procedures, and treatment options available to people who may be alcoholic or chemically dependent. The training also includes an examination of personal and group feelings and attitudes toward alcohol and drug issues, and an in-depth look at the dynamics of chemical dependency and its effects on families (COPES, 1998c).

The Developing Positive Parental Influences training promotes the skills of self-awareness and examines personal history and genetic risk factors. This enables people who are not already negatively involved with AOD to make responsible decisions regarding their AOD use behavior and to influence their children's

AOD use behaviors throughout their lives. The Developing Positive Parental Influences training focuses on separating thoughts and feelings along the continuum of abstinence, use, abuse, and dependency. It then shows how to apply these clarified thoughts and feelings in the area of behavioral standards for oneself and one's children based on familial, genetic, environment, and lifestyle risk factors (COPES, 1998c).

This training typically helps some participants recognize that they have significant levels of pain. For others, such pain is foreign to their experience. The pain some feel is associated with a broad range of personal or family experiences including family alcoholism, drunk driving crashes (in which there may have been fatalities), and a variety of other experiences. As this pain surfaces, some participants feel a need to process the pain, while others want to move on and focus on skill development or other aspects of the training. The trainers are encouraged to create an atmosphere of acceptance and inclusion of all participants in the training. This requires the facilitator to find an appropriate balance that includes allowing those in pain to express it and receive validation for it. It also includes moving beyond the personal tragedies with appropriate insight gained from these experiences for the larger group. Often some participants are unable to move beyond their own personal pain, and a referral to an outside treatment program is necessary. This allows the facilitator to step away from their personal issues without ignoring them and without allowing the group to become mired in one individual's personal tragedy.

Raising Resilient Youth Training

In addition to the general premises of CLFC provided earlier, the following premises are specific to the Raising Resilient Youth training:

1. Everyone needs feedback from others to know and improve themselves.
2. We teach and promote self-esteem in our children by listening to their thoughts and feelings with interest, respect, and understanding even when we disagree.
3. Children respond to opportunities to contribute to their family through responsible behavior only after years of practice.
4. Developing expectations and consequences is very different from setting rules and exacting punishments because the focus is on teaching and modeling responsibility rather than appearing to be retaliating for parental disappointment.
5. Children need and deserve unconditional love (i.e., no misbehavior can cause the absolute loss of love, respect, nurturance, support, or compassion) (COPES, 1998e).

This training allows parents to enhance their ability to develop and implement expectations and consequences with their children in many areas of interest and concern. Parents are taught how to include their children's active participation in setting expectations and consequences on a wide variety of issues important to the parent, including alcohol and drugs. This encourages dialogue, which in turn enhances a sense of competence, connectedness, and bonding between parent and child (COPES, 1998e).

The Raising Resilient Youth training operates under the overarching premise that it is possible for parents to learn more effective parenting knowledge, attitudes, and skills if they are given the opportunity to practice and test out these skills in a safe environment; and if practiced enough, these skills can become their natural way of responding to their children. In the Raising Resilient Youth training parents are exposed to the skills of expressing love, acceptance, and warmth for their children, negotiating healthy and positive expectations with their children, and consistently applying both positive and negative consequences for their children's positive and negative behaviors.

We have found that allowing the training to be accessed repeatedly helps some parents to better realize sustained behavioral change in their skills. We recommend that parents be given the opportunity to attend the Raising Resilient Youth Training as many times as necessary to practice effective parenting skills until they become confident of their ability to sustain these new parental skills.

Getting Real: A Communications Training for Parents, Youth, and Families

Some basic premises that are specific to the Getting Real Communications Training are as follows:

1. Communication is a deliberate attempt to impart one's ideas, feelings, desires, and beliefs.
2. Communication involves verbal and nonverbal messages (i.e., facial expressions, eye contact, and physical movements).
3. Communication is influenced by both conscious and unconscious thoughts and feelings.
4. By choosing to communicate clearly and express our feelings, we can increase the effectiveness of our interactions and enhance our relationships.
5. Being a good communicator takes practice and continued refinement of the various skills involved.
6. Being a good communicator involves being aware of the effect one's verbal and nonverbal responses have on others.

7. The responses we choose to use greatly influence how others will respond to us.
8. We can learn many things about ourselves by listening to others.
9. We can contribute to the growth of others by learning and using effective communication skills.
10. We can learn effective communication skills best in a group setting (COPES, 1998d, p. 12).

Human beings rely heavily on communication skills. Basic communication skills consist of listening, responding effectively, and both sending and receiving verbal and nonverbal messages. The Getting Real training operates under the primary rationale that communication is at its best when it establishes and maintains healthy, connected interpersonal relationships. A distinguishing feature of such relationships is that the parties involved know that their ideas and feelings are fully represented, validated, and respected.

The "Getting Real" communications module is a highly interactive training offered to both parents (and other caring adults) and youth who want to enhance their relationships by examining their responses to the verbal and nonverbal behavior they experience in their interactions with others. The following paragraphs draw extensively from COPES (1998d).

Through the Getting Real training, parents and youth learn to develop a greater awareness of the various types of responses (intimate and defensive), the various levels of communication, and the impact such factors have on the receiver of the communication. Participants are encouraged to enhance their personal communication through a three-step process: identify the response they most often use, examine their ability to express their feelings and ideas clearly, and establish a new pattern of interactions that will strengthen their relationships.

The Getting Real training is designed to promote the skills of self-awareness and mutual respect. It focuses on combining thoughts, feelings, and behavior in a way that leads the communicator to transmit powerful and meaningful messages. Finally, the training promotes insights and experiences that help us become effective listeners with others who may be struggling to say what they really want us to hear.

In the Getting Real training, participants focus on the two basic human reactions used in responding to both verbal and nonverbal behaviors of others. The two reactions are (1) intimate and (2) defensive, and they are basic human phenomena that cut across culture, class, education, and socioeconomic background.

Although there are six basic defensive responses, we find only one type of intimate response. We call this response "Getting Real." The Getting Real response is open, honest, clear, thoughtful, caring, and sensitive. It may also reveal the communicator's vulnerability. Getting Real can be an effective way to influence others. Although an intimate response may be given with varying degrees of depth, there is really only one type. It is sincere and authentic.

Defensive responses, however, are often controlling or manipulating. While they can be effective for the moment, they diminish closeness and intimacy in relationships over time. The list below identifies the common types of communication responses and the names we have given to each type:

The Intimate Response:

Open, honest, and respectful sharing of both thoughts and feelings	=	"Getting Real"

Defensive Responses:

Attacking	=	"Getting Rude"
Intellectualizing	=	"Getting Brainy"
Moralizing	=	"Getting Righteous"
Self-denial	=	"Giving In"
Avoiding	=	"Getting Away"
Joking	=	"Getting Funny"

Defensive responses often make people who use them feel good when they are using them and for a while after. However, they provide a false sense of well-being. For several minutes, hours, days, or weeks after using defensive responses, people may experience pain or regret for having used them. For example, defensive responses tend to have mixed effects. They

- Increase feelings of control, but result in loss of influence with others
- Increase a short-term sense of power, but result in loss of long-term power
- Increase a short-term sense of safety, but result in long-term loss of relationship and security
- Increase a short-term sense of pride, but result in long-term loss of self-esteem

Defensive responses decrease trust and respect for those who use them, and therefore also decrease one's positive influence with others. When we are defensive, we lose the opportunity to learn about ourselves from others. This results in low self-awareness, low self-improvement, and low potential for growth.

Through the Getting Real training, parents and youth are separated into their own peer groups and given the opportunity to learn about intimate and defensive responses through role-playing. The experiential (role-playing) nature of the training makes it fun and exciting for most participants. Since we know, however, that changing behaviors may also produce anxiety for some, Getting Real is designed to create an atmosphere of acceptance and comfort for everyone in the training, while simultaneously challenging participants to experience personal growth.

After parents learn these skills in the safety of their own peer groups, the adults and youth peer groups are brought together into a combined youth and adult Getting Real training to practice the skills together as family units.

The Getting Real training is effective in many critical areas:

- Increasing refusal skills
- Increasing a sense of internal locus of control
- Increasing self-efficacy
- Increasing self-worth
- Increasing self-respect
- Increasing respect for others
- Increasing the ability to gain the respect of others
- Enriching communication on an intimate level
- Increasing a sense of security
- Increasing family bonding

Training for Developing Independence and Responsibility

The Developing Independence and Responsibility training operates under the key premise that young people gain a deeper sense of fulfillment in their family life when they are treated with respect and expected to behave in a healthy, responsible, and developmentally appropriate manner. Other specific premises that guided the development of this training are as follows:

1. Young people often respond positively to high expectations.
2. Young people often feel validated and respected when they are asked to visualize themselves as successful and responsible adults in future years.
3. Responsibility, leadership, and cooperation are learned through years of practice.
4. Pain and powerlessness are natural and inevitable aspects of life.
5. Voluntary cooperation can be a source of satisfaction and closeness in a family.
6. Young people often respond positively to opportunities to contribute to the well-being of their family and community.
7. Young people often respond positively when they feel included in family discussions about expectations and consequences regarding their behavior (COPES, 1998b, p. 10).

In this training, youth are asked to examine their current level of personal responsibility in their family life, with an eye toward developing personal independence and responsibility for adulthood. The following description of this training module draws extensively from COPES (1998b).

Using activities similar to those in the Raising Resilient Youth training for parents, we ask youth to visualize themselves in roles such as future parents, co-workers, supervisors, or other adults responsible for setting appropriate expectations and consequences for their children or others they may supervise in areas of responsibility.

This technique has proven useful for several reasons. Youth are often frustrated by feelings of powerlessness, domination, and even low self-esteem when they find themselves at the receiving end of rules, expectations, and consequences. In this training design, we encourage youth to visualize themselves in a more equalitarian or even upper-handed position of power and influence.

This visualizing exercise helps them to recognize their potential and affirm their sense of self-esteem. It provides them with concrete evidence that we (the adult world), through our expectations that youth will rise to positions of power and influence in later years, do recognize their value, power, and worth. As the youth struggle with the difficulties of parental and supervisory roles, their sensitivity toward parents and other adults who supervise them is increased. Many young people find themselves helpfully challenged when we ask them about the expectations they would place on their children regarding alcohol and drugs, violent behavior, curfews, chores, schoolwork, bedtimes, and other day-to-day issues in their lives.

Ultimately, participating youth often recognize and appreciate the difficulties their parents currently face within the context of their family. When their parents are simultaneously engaged in the Raising Resilient Youth training, a more productive level of household dialogue generally occurs, enhancing a family's sense of connectedness, competence, and parent and youth bonding.

Developing a Positive Response:
An Alcohol and Drug Training for Youth

The basic premises on which the Developing a Positive Response training was developed are as follows:

1. Independence does not come without responsibility.
2. Responsibility is learned through practice.
3. Respect is learned by receiving it.
4. Extreme attitudes and behaviors are dangerous because they promote both themselves and their opposites.

5. Pain is a natural part of life. It is normal to feel pain.
6. When a person hurts, it helps to express feelings (COPES, 1998a, p. 10).

The Developing a Positive Response training component (COPES, 1998a) is designed to encourage youth to examine their knowledge, attitudes, beliefs, and skills regarding AOD use issues. This training seeks to help young people become aware of hopes for their own personal health, their relationships with their peers and family members, and their desires for success. Through this training, youth build the foundation for increasing their skills in communicating their deepest wishes about AOD issues with their family and friends and are helped to recognize their growing (and developmentally appropriate) yearnings for independence from the negative pressures and negative behaviors in their social environments (COPES, 1998a). These skills are reinforced through two other training modules, the youth Developing Independence and Responsibility training and the Getting Real Communications Training, discussed in a previous section. Further, these skills are increased within the family domain through their parents' participation in the parent training modules. Together these learning experiences help youth to recognize that their decisions regarding AOD use do matter, and the program equips them for making healthy decisions that increase their likelihood of success.

The Developing a Positive Response training is intended for implementation with youth between the ages of 9 and 17. Because of developmental differences, however, it is helpful to implement the training with youth who are within age-appropriate groupings. These age groupings are 9 to 11, 12 to 14, and 15 to 17.

We believe that youth develop appropriate alcohol- and drug-related values and beliefs when the adults in their lives model them. Modeling of these values and beliefs is therefore important for those who facilitate the Developing a Positive Response module. In addition, the parent training module on alcohol and drugs (Developing Positive Parental Influences) is designed to assist the parent in modeling behaviors that manifest these beliefs. When parents and other adults are perceived as living models of these values and beliefs, youth receive the support and guidance they need to develop appropriate independence and autonomy. Even when a child's parent is incapable of modeling healthy behaviors after the program ends, their children have been exposed in the training to other adults who *are* successful in doing so. This limited exposure to other appropriate adult role models seems to help some young people to realize their yearnings for success, health, and self-esteem in decision making regarding AOD and other personal health issues.

Being exposed to the facilitator (a healthy adult model) and other healthy parents often proves to be a strong contributing factor to the healthy development of children whose parents struggle in their own lives with appropriate behavior. In Chapter 6, we will discuss the importance of well-equipped, nurturing, and effective trainers who can model the essence of the CLFC training premises in their everyday lives. In addition, we will describe the process used by COPES to assess and prepare potential CLFC trainers.

In the next chapter, we will present specific examples from three CLFC training modules. These will provide the reader a greater understanding of how the CLFC program components play out in actual communities among actual participants.

4

Illustrative Examples from the Parent and Youth Training Components

In this chapter, we will present examples of specific training exercises used in the CLFC parent and youth trainings. By exploring these illustrative exercises and reviewing typical experiences that occur during the implementation of the exercises, the reader will get a clearer sense of how the program plays out in local communities.

THE PERSONAL EXPERIENCES WITH ALCOHOL EXERCISE FROM THE DEVELOPING POSITIVE PARENTAL INFLUENCES TRAINING

The Personal Experiences with Alcohol exercise illustrates the types of training that participants experience in the adult alcohol and drug issues training sessions. This exercise is the initial activity of the Developing Positive Parental Influences training (COPES, 1998c). At the start, participants are asked to recall the first time, if ever, they had a drink of alcohol, and the first time, if ever, they became drunk. They are asked to remember where they were, how old they were, and their thoughts and feelings at the time. The trainer then shares his or her first drink story and first drunk story. This gives participants a chance to hear one person's story, which triggers their own personal memories before they are asked to share their story with the group. Additionally, the trainer models an appropriate level of openness for participants to follow.

It is important for trainers to provide detailed recollections of their experiences and to discuss especially the feelings associated with these events. A typical trainer's story might go something like this:

> I was reared in the South; smack dab in the middle of the Bible Belt. My father's family was Baptist and my mother's family was Methodist. Because of this, drinking was considered to be immoral by my immediate family. My grandfather on my father's side was an alcoholic. I do not remember him drinking, because he had stopped drinking before I was old enough to remember. Because of the pain that my father experienced from my grandfather's alcoholism, he was a strict "abstainer." He would not even allow alcohol in his home. The only prevention message I received from him about drinking was, "If I ever catch you drinking, I will kill you!"
>
> I was 18 years old before I ever tried alcohol, which was the legal drinking age at the time. I was with friends. I had a boat and spent most of the summer on the lake near our house boating and camping. I had three or four friends that I hung out with every day. However, this one guy had infiltrated my small circle of friends. I knew he was pretty wild, yet the other guys liked him so I pretended to like him too. One day he stated that he knew where we could get some beer. I did not want to get any, but everyone else did so I went along with the group. Peer pressure, I guess.
>
> We went to a boat dock up the lake and we got two six packs of beer. It was getting late, so we took the beer back to our campsite, built a fire, and we sat around the fire and began to drink it. The first time I tasted it, I was scared. I remember thinking, "If my father is so worried about me drinking, then what is this stuff going to do to me? Is it going to make me crazy?" But I felt pressured to try it, so I did. It tasted nasty. I hated it. Yet I pretended to like it so the others guys wouldn't think I was a geek. When no one was looking, I would pour it out to make it look like I was actually drinking it. I was convinced that the other guys were pouring theirs out too because there was no way they could drink this nasty stuff. I did not drink enough for it to have any effect on me and I don't remember any of the other guys acting crazy either.
>
> Soon this became the thing to do. Every time we were in the boat, we would get beer. By the end of the summer, I actually got to a point where I could drink three or four. The first time I remember feeling drunk was one day late in the summer. I drank about four or five beers along with the rest of my friends. I remember feeling excited, daring, bold, and powerful. We decided to play this game called Figure

Eight. To play this game, a person would get in the tube tied behind the boat, and someone would drive the boat in a figure eight. The person who could stay on the tube the longest won. Of course, we were feeling daring and cocky so we were all thinking we could stay on the tube without falling off. One of my friends jumped on the tube and stated that there was no way we could throw him off. I was driving the boat. Of course, I felt challenged by that statement. I started going really fast in a figure eight motion. My friend on the tube was going so fast that he would pass up the boat in the turns. While he was riding the tube, he was yelling. We thought he was yelling for us to go faster. So I did. I slung him around like crazy. At times the only thing on the tube was the arm with which he was holding on. Finally, we determined that he was in trouble. He had placed his hand in the rope that was tied to the tube with a slipknot. The faster I went the tighter the rope got on his hand. Before we stopped, the rope had crushed his hand.

We had to rush him to the hospital. He had to have several surgeries on his hand, and it never fully recovered. Our parents found out that we were drunk. The only thing my father said to me was, "I never thought a son of mine would ever do that." Several months passed before he even spoke to me after that day. So my first drunk was exciting at first, but I ended up feeling responsible for my friend's injury, ashamed, embarrassed, and rejected by my father.

After the trainers share their personal stories (like the example above), participants are encouraged to share their personal experiences with alcohol. It is expected that all trainers will tell their own personal story as it actually occurred. It is not necessary that there be a negative or serious consequence resulting from the inappropriate use of alcohol. Unfortunately, some trainers feel compelled to overemphasize negative consequences so as to clearly convey their stance against alcohol abuse. However, such embellishment will probably not ring true to the participants. Trainers will have ample opportunity to express their personal convictions later in the training. Trainers who tell the story as it actually occurred are perceived as much less manipulative by the participants.

We remind participants to tell the group who they were with and how old they were at the time, and to report their honest thoughts and feelings to the best of their recollection. We also remind participants that the trainers have shared their stories many times and have thus been able to recollect a lot of detail. We reassure participants that their stories are not expected to be as elaborate as the trainers' stories. In addition, we remind participants about confidentiality rules and the right to pass if they do not want to share. As participants share their stories, trainers attempt to elicit more information or feelings, if necessary.

SOME KEY LEARNING OBJECTIVES OF THE PERSONAL EXPERIENCES WITH ALCOHOL EXERCISE

After participants share their personal experiences, the trainers process the stories with the group. What follows are some key learning objectives that are targeted through this activity.

1. Trainers seek to learn as much as possible about the participants' personal and family history, religious beliefs, and beliefs and attitudes toward drinking, drunkenness, and alcoholism. This helps them gain a better understanding of participants' frames of reference for this and the other CLFC training modules. Just by hearing the sample story provided here, one can glean much information: (a) the trainer came from a religious background that viewed drinking as an immoral act, (b) his grandfather was an alcoholic, (c) his father was the child of an alcoholic, (d) his family held extreme attitudes and beliefs about drinking, (e) his parents did not discuss expectations and consequences about drinking in an appropriate manner, and (f) he learned the "ground rules" of drinking from his friends, not his parents.
2. Religious beliefs can have a powerful influence on someone's attitudes toward drinking.
3. Family attitudes have a powerful influence on one's personal beliefs and attitudes, especially on extreme attitudes. Possessing extreme attitudes often causes a person to lose influence. For example, the trainer's father said he would kill him if he ever caught him drinking. Obviously, it is easy for a young person to dismiss such a threat as an unthinkable consequence. Extreme messages, such as "alcohol will kill you," can also be easily dismissed when young people see others drinking without any problems.
4. Many young people drink before the legal drinking age. Often participants disclose that they were as young as 7 or 8 when they had their first drink. Therefore, it is important for parents to begin early discussing expectations regarding drinking.
5. There are many similarities and differences among participants. Most participants report that they were under the legal drinking age when they first tried alcohol. Most often, participants were with friends the first time they got drunk. Many were exposed to their first drink by their parents. It is common for participants to struggle with naming feelings. It is common for several of the participants to have family members who suffer from alcoholism.

6. It is important to be clear about the language we use when discussing these events. Participants often use the word "drinking" when they are in fact discussing drunkenness or alcoholism.

7. Often children are left to learn about drinking from their friends. In the narrative in this chapter, the trainer's friends taught him that drinking is a rite of passage and that the more one can drink, the more "macho" one is. These are clearly not the messages a young person should receive about drinking.

8. It is important to recognize, name, and express feelings. In the sample story, if the trainer had been able to discuss his feelings with his friends and stand up for his beliefs, then he would not have experienced the negative consequences of bad decisions.

The authors have conducted this exercise with thousands of people in the United States. Virtually any group of more than 10 parents is likely to provide a genuine cross section of experiences. Most but not all adults have tasted alcohol. Many but not all who have tasted alcohol have experienced at least some level of intoxication. Many have dealt with alcoholism within their own family. Some are already worried about what their children see in their own family and community environment. Some are themselves recovering alcoholics. All appear to want their children to avoid alcoholism. We can learn a lot from other people's stories. Participants discover that we all grow up with different beliefs and experiences relating to alcohol. Participants also discover that the way we react to alcohol and what we have come to expect from it have much to do with what we saw and heard about alcohol as children. Virtually all of the adults who participate in this exercise begin to take their role as parents more seriously after listening to a group of other adults talk about their first-drink/first-drunk experiences.

We now consider some of the common elements of the first-drink stories we regularly hear in this exercise. For many, the first drink occurs at home, between the ages of 10 and 20, with appropriate information, guidance, and support. For these people, a typical reaction involves a sense of inclusion, acceptance, and satisfaction of curiosity. The greatest number typically are surprised by the realization that they do not like the taste.

For others, the first drink occurs in their late teens, in secret, with peers. Often these individuals come from abstaining families where it may even be considered a sin to drink. These participants often report that they reacted to their first drink experience with fear, excitement, and guilt.

For still others, the first drink occurs before age 10, is taken at home (often from a parent's liquor supply), in secret and alone. They report that they did it out of personal curiosity, often because there was little open discussion within their family regarding alcohol use. Many report that this first experience was shocking, painful (i.e., burning), and confusing.

Let's now consider some of the common elements of the first drunk stories we hear in this exercise. For most, their first drunk occurs in a peer setting, just as it did in the trainer's story above. Also, for most, a number of years pass between first drink and first drunk. For some, the first-drink episode includes several drinks, and becomes the first-drunk episode as well. Also, for most, the first-drunk episode includes excitement, some pleasure, and some unexpected sickness and/or a variety of other negative consequences. Much less frequently, the first-drunk episode is reported as being fun, pleasurable, and lacking any recognized negative consequences. Many other people have simply never experienced intoxication at all.

It is interesting to correlate the details of first-drink and first-drunk stories with what participants are telling each other about their personal family environment regarding alcohol use, abuse, and dependency. In the general discussion that follows the sharing of these stories, many parents appear very thoughtful about what they now want to tell their children and about what they show their children through their behavior. For example, very few parents who drink continue to do so without engaging in some very specific dialogue with their children about the role alcohol should or should not play in their children's lives. Also, abstaining families seem to find it useful to talk in new ways to their children about how they may be exposed to alcohol with their peers as they reach the teenage years.

Overall, through this exercise parents begin to recognize their own desire to educate their children in more deliberate ways. Moreover, they do so without having received a lecture from the facilitator on what to do and how to do it. Creating exercises where adults are affirmed as being the major decision makers for their own family is most beneficial in reducing resistance to parent programming. No facilitator should be put in the position of spouting a single approach for all parents to adopt. Yet when exercises such as this one are handled properly, most parent participants reach supportable conclusions without engaging in any power struggles or enduring a pedantic lecture that leaves the whole group in discomfort. The facilitator is subtly modeling a nonjudgmental and accepting approach to both abstainers and those who choose to drink alcohol in low-risk ways. The two extreme positions—alcohol is great, the more the better; and abstinence with a vengeance—rarely find much support in the overall group. Their extreme nature carry obvious complications that are easily recognized by the larger group on reflection. It is to be noted that abstinence without a punitive attitude is not considered an extreme position.

We next examine the Feelings exercise, a skill-building exercise in the Raising Resilient Youth training

THE FEELINGS EXERCISE

Below is a copy of the handout given to parents who participate in this exercise. You may want to fill it out for yourself now, so that as you read the chapter, you can have a vicarious experience of the group exercise.

Handout for Feelings Exercise

We believe it is important for parents and other caring adults to be able to recognize and name feelings and be able to listen to and affirm others' feelings as they arise in everyday situations. Emotions or feelings are an important part of the process of developing expectations, rules, and consequences for your child. The following exercise is designed to provide adults with an opportunity to examine how they each might feel in certain situations and to check their feelings vocabularies. There are no right or wrong answers. Simply list what you might feel in these situations. **Following this exercise is a feelings vocabulary list. Feel free to use it to locate those feelings that are hard to name.**

Each parent and/or other significant adult in the family should attempt to list three emotions he or she might feel in the following situations. Each person works on their own list individually, without discussing the situations. Later you will be asked to share your personal responses for comparison and discussion.

Here is a list of fictional situations in which people might find themselves. Please list three emotions **you** might experience in each of these situations.

1. Everyone joined in cleaning the house and it looks great.
   List three feelings you might have _____ _____ _____

2. In the middle of the night your telephone rings. A male, adult-sounding voice says, "I am sorry to tell you that your child has been involved in an accident." There is a pause, so you say, "Oh no, what happened?" The voice says, "Fifteen years ago tonight your child wet the bed." He laughs and hangs up.
   List three feelings you might have _____ _____ _____

3. You are driving a long distance on your vacation. Two hundred miles from your destination, you encounter stalled traffic on the interstate. The last exit was five miles back. Up ahead you see police vehicles, flashing lights and several people crowded at the front of the stalled traffic line.
   List three feelings you might have _____ _____ _____

4. A good friend tells you she is moving to California in the following week to care for her ailing and extremely wealthy grandmother. It is apparent your friend has been planning this move for quite some time, but she says she didn't know how to tell you until now.
   List three feelings you might have _____ _____ _____

5. Your teenager has a curfew for 11:00 p.m. on weekends. It is Saturday night at 12:30 a.m. and your teenager is not home yet and has not called to explain why he or she is late.
   List three feelings you might have _____ _____ _____

6. While you are out working in the yard, your next door neighbor runs out of her house. She is bleeding from her lower lip. She runs to you, grasps your arm and says, "He's done this before. But promise me one thing. You won't tell anyone about this or the other times, no matter what, OK?"
   List three feelings you might have _____ _____ _____

7. At Wal-Mart, your child has been hassling you to purchase something for him. Repeatedly you refuse. The situation escalates until the child is wailing uncontrollably, to the obvious discomfort of the other shoppers.
   List three feelings you might have _____ _____ _____

8. While watching the lottery drawing on TV, you realize that you have the winning numbers. You go to the kitchen counter to get the ticket and discover it is no longer there. You frantically ask everyone if they have seen it. Your teenager states that she thought it was an old one and threw it away.
   List three feelings you might have _____ _____ _____

9. You have been offered a new job with a substantial increase in salary. In order to accept the new job, you must be willing to relocate.
   List three feelings you might have _____ _____ _____

10. You have left your only child at home with a neighbor's daughter in order to attend an important social gathering downtown. At 1:30 a.m. you turn down your street and see fire trucks in front of your house. Your child and the sitter are nowhere to be found. Moments later, the sitter drives up in another car. You see your child is safe. You ask, "What happened?" The sitter says, "I don't know. I went to visit a friend and I stayed a little later than I planned. I'm sorry. I thought I'd get back before you did."
    List three feelings you might have _____ _____ _____

11. As a single parent, you have recently begun dating a new person. Your children, who have not met your new friend yet, express a desire to meet him/her.
    List three feelings you might have _____ _____ _____

12. A new family moved into the house next door. Your children become friends with their children, who are about the same age. You begin to notice that your children always seem to have something new when coming from the neighbor's house.
    List three feelings you might have _____ _____ _____

13. Your child has just graduated from high school with honors. She has received a scholarship to attend a prestigious college in New England.
    List three feelings you might have _____ _____ _____

14. You've had a stressful day at work. You come home to lots of chores. Your six-year-old wants your immediate attention to show you his schoolwork.
    List three feelings you might have _____ _____ _____

15. You're going to a family gathering for Thanksgiving dinner. You'll be reunited with some relatives whom you haven't seen for years.
    List three feelings you might have _____ _____ _____

16. Your mother calls. She says she hasn't been feeling well and may need an operation.
    List three feelings you might have _____ _____ _____

17. You're in the mall and you notice that the sales clerk has waited on someone who came in after you.
    List three feelings you might have _____ _____ _____

Feelings Vocabulary List

Glad	Caring	Sad	Confused	Hurt		Mad	
Glad	Liking	Unhappy	Uncertain	Neglected	Miffed	Mad	
Contented	Friendliness	Disappointed	Dubious	Discounted	Irked	Aggravated	
Satisfied	Fondness	Glum	Unsure	Disappointed	Perturbed	Vexed	
Calm	Regard	Bored	Uncomfortable	Envious	Chagrined	Vindictive	
Cheerful	Sympathy	Distressed	Undecided	Frustrated	Cross	Furious	
Pleased	Respect	Apathetic	Troubled	Abused	Dismayed	Enraged	
Serene	Empathy	Sorrowful	Frustrated	Deprecated	Impatient	Seething	
Joyful	Admiring	Discouraged	Disturbed	Disparaged	Resentful	Outraged	
Ecstatic	Concern	Melancholy	Ambivalent	Scorned	Irritated	Infuriated	
Excited	Trust	Depressed	Bewildered	Used	Hostile	Indignant	
Elated	Closeness	Desolated	Baffled	Exploited	Annoyed	Bitter	
Exhilarated	Affection	Dejected	Trapped	Debased	Agitated		
Euphoric	Love	Hopeless		In pain			
Enthusiastic	Devotion	Gloomy		Devastated			
Delighted	Pity	Dismal		Humiliated			
	Attachment	Despairing		Anguished			
		Empty		Rejected			
		Grieving					

Lonely	Guilt-Shame	Interest	Inadequate	Adequate		Fear	
Lonesome	Regretful	Curious	Unsure	Sure	Nervous	Scared	
Alienated	Embarrassed	Captivated	Uncertain	Certain	Apprehensive	Anxious	
Remote	Responsible	Interested	Cautious	Confident	Timid	Defensive	
Alone	Ashamed	Eager	eak	Strong	Shy	Intimidated	
Isolated	Guilty	Challenged	Defeated	Capable	Worried	Dreading	
Abandoned	Remorseful	Fascinated	Jealous	Powerful	Uneasy	Desperate	
	Humiliated	Inspired	Overwhelmed	Competent	Bashful	Frantic	
			Worthless	Useful	Uncomfortable	Panic	
			Powerless	Proud	Afraid	Terror	
			Helpless	Brave	Frightened		
			Inferior	Daring			
			Useless	Bold			
				Superior			

How the Feelings Exercise Might Play Out

In the Personal Experiences with Alcohol exercise described earlier in this chapter, we presented a sample story that a trainer might use in the exercise and a narrative summary regarding how it plays out in a training. For the Feelings exercise, we will describe what a typical exercise might be like and draw the reader vicariously into an actual training section.

Imagine that you (and perhaps your spouse) have just completed filling out the above exercise by listing three feelings *for each scenario.* To experience the full effect of this exercise, please do so now before reading any further. Now imagine that you are in a group training session with other parents. The facilitator asks the group, "How did it *feel* to answer these questions?" No one speaks up for a moment or two. Then Shirley, a 35-year-old mother of two, replies in an unusually cheerful tone, "I think this was fun!" Immediately, a large and usually quiet man named Bill hisses out a heavy sigh and visibly rolls his eyes in an apparent response to her comment.

You're sitting there and you and everyone else knows the facilitator heard and saw both reactions. The facilitator pauses thoughtfully before saying anything, and everyone sits in silence. Finally the facilitator looks warmly at Bill and says, "I'm just guessing, Bill, but I'm betting this wasn't fun for you, and I'm just wondering if you're thinking about how ridiculous this whole business is?" Bill doesn't respond verbally, yet he changes his sitting posture and adjusts his shirt collar. The young mother, Shirley, is scanning the group in what appears to be an attempt to assess the group's level of support in seeing this as "fun." The facilitator speaks up again, "Well, Bill, let me tell you that I have conducted this exercise with a large number of groups, and these groups are made up of a lot of very unique individuals. I see a wide variety of reactions to this exercise, and to every question in this exercise. Some people really like it, and some people think it is a total waste of time. And you know what? Both perceptions are exactly correct. Now I'm not suggesting, Bill, that you believe this exercise is a complete waste of time, I'm just saying I wouldn't be surprised if you or someone else in this group did react that way. Yet I am curious—are you going to tell me your reaction to it? My curiosity was triggered by what sounded like a plaintive sigh escaping from you just as Shirley said this was fun."

The facilitator pauses in silence, awaiting a response. Finally Bill says, "No, no, I liked it all okay. It's only that I just remembered I was supposed to pick up my daughter on my way here from work and I forgot. I've got to go."

He raises himself out of his chair and walks toward the door. As Bill is leaving, the facilitator says, "Bill, I know I hate it when I forget that kind of stuff, and I'm really glad that you remembered now before its too late. Good luck and I hope to see you next week!"

Bill responds, "Oh, I'll be back shortly, I hope."

"Great—I hope to see you soon then." Then the facilitator turns to the group again and says, "Well, what are you thinking and feeling now?" As the facilitator is asking this, it appears to you that she is looking at you personally for some sort of response.

You are formulating a response when another young father says, "I'm thinking it's a good thing that guy remembered his daughter when he did. I hope he finds her and everything is okay." A general sense of agreement exudes from the group, and the facilitator responds, "I want to continue this exercise on thinking and feeling and also talk a little more about what just happened to this gentleman who suddenly realized that he forgot to get his daughter. He seemed to be hit with some feelings and thought that required some action or behavior. It was just like one of the examples from the list of situations in this exercise. In each of these 17 situations in this exercise we find ourselves confronted with something that might impact our emotions, engage our thinking, and lead to some behavior, right?" The group nods in agreement.

"Also, in many of these situations there may be other people who might also have their own separate emotions and thoughts that might influence their actions too, right?" Again, general agreement comes from the group.

"Well, in this training program, we believe it is helpful for people to identify and share their thoughts and their feelings before jumping into any active or reactive behavior. Sometimes it can be very helpful for a person to get a sense of everyone else's thoughts and feelings, too, before choosing his next action. When he is able to understand both his own and other people's thoughts and feelings, he is in a very powerful position to manage his decisions regarding his actions and behavior. Finally, many people find it rewarding and reassuring to feel listened to and affirmed by others with regard to how they are reacting emotionally to a situation."

"So now, together, let's review several of these situations in the exercise and examine how we each respond using feelings words. Let's compare a few individual responses and let's also try to affirm all the different emotional responses that each of us might have had. In doing so, I believe we can learn about ourselves and about others, and how we can affirm each other in our relationships."

After that brief lecture, the facilitator asks for volunteers to share their personal lists of three feelings words that might describe their reactions. The facilitator listens to and personally affirms each feelings reaction shared voluntarily. At the same time, the facilitator listens for nonaffirming reactions from other participants as the volunteer reads his or her list of feelings words. Nonaffirming reactions come in many varieties. A few examples are listed here:

How could you feel that way?
You shouldn't feel like that.
That's weird!
You're crazy!
What!?

If a participant reacts to another's feelings response with a nonaffirming reaction, the facilitator openly examines with both participants the effect this might have on their "relationship." By doing so, it often becomes clear how nonaffirming reactions to other people's feelings create increased pain, decreased relationships, decreased support, lowered self-esteem, and increased conflict.

Some Key Learning Objectives of the Feelings Exercise

While participants usually enjoy the discussion involving a wide variety of emotional reactions to these situations, it also helps them recognize some important social dynamics. The facilitator attempts to elicit group recognition and discussion of the following points:

1. There are many similar reactions among group members, and this is affirming for those participants having similar reactions.
2. There are also individual reactions that may be very different from those of others. These people deserve and enjoy affirmation too. A simple nod or comment that says "Oh, I see how you could feel that way" is very helpful.
3. When we affirm how others feel, our relationships and bonding are strengthened and our "influence" with people is increased.
4. Recognizing and naming our feelings and gaining affirmation of those feelings before choosing to act or react can be beneficial. This prevents impulsive reactions, which often add to the likelihood of ongoing problems.
5. Recognition and awareness of our emotional reaction to a situation and sharing this information with others often leads to good decisions about how to respond to a challenging situation.
6. If someone notices that a single major feeling dominates her own list of responses in this exercise (like anger or frustration), it may suggest that this is something to think about more deeply. Some people develop "emotional habits of response," a sort of one-feeling-fits-almost-all-situations reaction. Some people (and their families) find it refreshing to notice these habits and to begin to open their minds to discovering more varied and rich patterns of response. This is usually both challenging and rewarding for everyone involved.

After all of these observations have either been discovered by the group or introduced and explored by the facilitator, the exercise can move toward conclusion.

The Feelings Exercise Concluded

Having reviewed some of the key points provided in the Feelings exercise, let's tune back in as our facilitator concludes the session.

"Now let's return to our experience with Bill at the beginning of our exercise. Here he is sitting in this training session, reading about all these little situations that might trigger some emotions, and all of a sudden real life intrudes as he remembers that he was supposed to pick up his daughter. What happened first?"

Shirley jumps in, "Well, he sighed, and I thought he was reacting to me saying this was fun."

"Yes, what was that like for you?"

"Well, I guess I felt defensive, like he was putting me down!"

The facilitator says, "Yes, I know, I suspected that too. I even almost said so, but I also tried to just tell him my thoughts and feelings and see if your perceptions and mine were correct."

"So, what do you suppose the sigh was expressing?"

Shirley suggests, "Bill was probably frustrated or irritated that he had forgotten her."

Another participant suggests, "I think he was embarrassed about interrupting the group and by having to leave."

The facilitator says, "Well, it seems obvious that some emotion was trying to escape to the light of day, huh? So then he expressed the situation, and I tried to affirm him and support his decision to leave. I was worried that he or the group might think that I would be upset if he left. You know, like I'm the facilitator and you can't leave without a note from the teacher sort of thing?"

"Well, maybe next time we'll see if Bill can tell us his exact feelings. As a matter of fact, I'm feeling a little bit worried because he didn't come back, did he?" Many participants look around. Some seem to have expressions of worry while others are smiling and joking, and still others are getting their things in preparation to leave.

"Well, I hope to see all of you next week, and I hope Bill can give us the rest of the story."

EXAMPLE FROM THE GETTING REAL MODULE

The Getting Real Communication Module is a highly interactive training offered to parents, youth, and other caring adults interested in enhancing their relationships by examining their responses to the verbal and nonverbal behavior they experience in their interactions with others. The training can be implemented for families in two ways:

- Option 1: Provide only the separate parent and youth peer component (four to five sessions).
- Option 2: Provide both the separate parent and youth peer components (four to five sessions) and the parent and youth combined component (two to three sessions) for a total of six to eight sessions.

Participants in the Getting Real training are expected to develop a greater awareness of the various types of communication responses (both intimate and defensive) through role plays, understanding the various levels of communication, and discovering the impact such factors have on the receiver of the communication.

All participants are encouraged to enhance their personal communication by (1) identifying the response they use most, (2) examining their ability to express their feelings and ideas clearly, and (3) establishing a new pattern of interactions that will enrich their relationships. Getting Real training promotes skills of self-awareness and mutual respect. It focuses on combining thoughts, feelings, and behavior in a way that leads the communicator to transmit the message more meaningfully. Finally, the training promotes insights and experiences that help us to become great listeners to others who may be struggling to say what they really want us to hear.

The Getting Real Training Model

The Getting Real training is powerful for both adults and youth. However, for it to be most relevant, comfortable, and effective for the participants, it is necessary to provide most of the training for adults and youth separately. This training involves the enactment of situations in which we may see, hear, and fully experience the behavior of others in a safe setting (role play). Adults experience role playing in very different ways than young people. For that reason, this training is most helpful when it is first provided to adults and youth separately.

Getting Real—Peer Component

Once the group of adults and youth have been divided into their peer groups, the trainer should use the training manual and the accompanying posters to facilitate the training process.

The training manual also provides several examples of age-appropriate situations (role plays) that have been helpful in illustrating the intimate and defensive responses. As facilitators gain experience and confidence, they often decide to enact role plays that have been suggested in discussions with participants. Situations should involve one person pressuring another person to do or discuss something that he or she has a reason to resist. The responses are best illustrated when used to deal with social pressure or discomfort of some kind.

Role plays, based on posters and other situations provided in the manual, serve as an important instructional tool within this training model. Each participant will benefit from the opportunity to participate in at least two role plays and the training facilitator can be instrumental in ensuring that this happens. The role-play experience provides participants with an opportunity to:

- Explore their own thoughts, feelings, verbal responses, and nonverbal responses
- Receive feedback from others about their ability to respond effectively
- Practice intimate responses
- See peers demonstrate the various responses
- Recognize the difference between intimate and defensive responses

It may be necessary to ask participants who volunteer repeatedly to allow others the opportunity to participate. It may also be necessary to gently encourage participation from those who are reluctant to participate. Perhaps most important, the trainer can facilitate maximum participation by creating a training environment in which each participant's rights (including the right to pass) are respected.

The intimate and defensive responses represented in this training model, which were described in Chapter 3, are basic human phenomena that transcend culture, class, and educational and socioeconomic background. However, be alert for nuances that may be unique to your group. You may find that the youth develop these skills much more quickly than the adults. Adults are typically more comfortable with the pattern of responses they have developed over a long period of time, and may thus find it difficult to change old habits. The youth, on the other hand, integrate the skills more quickly because they have not yet developed an entrenched set of defensive responses.

Next, let's look at one sample situation that occurred in an adult Getting Real training session.

In the adult Getting Real training, adult volunteers are asked to participate in a role-playing situation. Sometimes, the facilitator will begin the session with the situation (scenario) depicted on the sample posters provided in the training materials. Let's examine two of these posters, "The Situation" (Figure 4.1) and "When Giving In" (Figure 4.2).

Figure 4.1 is a poster that depicts a man pressing someone to contribute money to a fund-raising effort. This role play requires two volunteers. One volunteer will assume this pressuring role, while the other will be asked to respond to the pressure using two different response styles in two separate role plays. Each role-play volunteer is also asked to select a name from another poster that has a list of "stage names." In our example the male volunteer selects the stage name "Elvis Priestly." The facilitator reviews this person's expected role and encourages "Elvis" to pressure the other volunteer into giving a contribution during the role play.

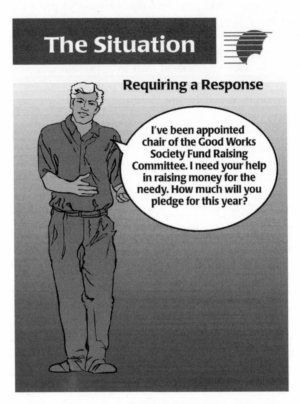

Figure 4.1.

The second volunteer, a woman who selects the stage name "Reba McIntosh," is asked to review the "When Giving In" poster (Figure 4.2). The man on the poster is shown to be *thinking:* "I don't want to give. I'm short of cash." He is illustrated as *feeling:* "I'm angry and irritated. I feel pressured! I want to keep you as a friend." Yet he is *saying:* "Yes, I'll be glad to contribute to the fund-raising effort."

The facilitator again reviews the situation and illustrates the "Giving In" response.

FACILITATOR: Have you ever been pressured by someone and ended up saying yes when you would have honestly preferred to say no? Well, we would like for you, under your stage name, to show us what this might look like in real life by playing this Giving In role in a role play here with Elvis. Let's make it fun now—don't just say yes. Show us a few attempts at light resistance so Elvis has to work at it. Reba, are you ready?

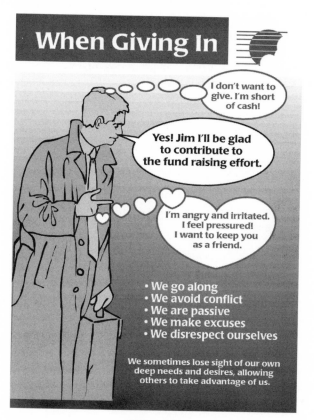

Figure 4.2.

REBA: I think so.

FACILITATOR: Elvis?

ELVIS: (pulls up his shirt collar and speaks in a pseudo Elvis Presley voice) Yeah, man I'm ready; thank you, thank you very much! [The rest of the participants laugh.]

FACILITATOR: (turns to the group) OK, that's good. All of you now are the audience for this role play. And you've got a job to do as well. Your job is to observe this role play and look for three things.

The facilitator then points to a poster titled Audience Instructions which reads as follows:

1. Study our role players' body movements.
2. Look for respect and friendship between these two.
3. Identify what you might have wanted to see happen.

FACILITATOR: Is that clear to everyone? Okay, then, if our role players are still ready? Okay. Ready, set, go.

ELVIS: Now, Reba, I've got a hard job here, and I really need your help with a little ten-dollar donation for needy children.

REBA: Oh, I don't know, Elvis, I'm pretty low on cash.

ELVIS: I understand, Reba, but I bought two raffle tickets from you when you were selling them for your children's choir, didn't I? Come on, it's just ten bucks. You can pay me back later. I'll put it in for you now and you can get me ten dollars on payday next week. Okay? . . .

REBA: My kids' tickets were only one dollar. Come on, Elvis, really. I don't know if I can handle it!

ELVIS: Well, Reba, no big deal. Like I said, I'll just put it in here for you now and you can pay me back later, okay? Come on, Reba, this is for needy kids and surely you can handle ten bucks. Gosh, it's not that much.

REBA: Well, I guess so, Elvis, but don't be in any big hurry to collect, okay?

ELVIS: Okay! It's a deal!

FACILITATOR: Okay—Cut. Great job! Now let's talk about this folks. First of all, Elvis, what was this like for you?

ELVIS: This was fun. I got Reba there to give me ten bucks.

FACILITATOR: Tell me what you were thinking about.

ELVIS: Well, I was thinking that I had to get the money.

FACILITATOR: How did you feel about what you said and did?

ELVIS: Successful! I mean I got her to do it, right?

FACILITATOR: Well, yes, but tell me, Elvis, about your sense of closeness or intimacy with Reba. Do you feel close to her now?

ELVIS: Well, let's see—no, not really close or anything, but hey, I got the money.

FACILITATOR: Okay, now tell me about your sense of self-respect.

ELVIS: Well, it's okay. I got the money.

FACILITATOR: Yes, and do you like the way you did it?

ELVIS: I don't know.

FACILITATOR: Well, do you feel good about how you did it? You know, I'm not sure she really wanted to do it.

ELVIS: Well, my job was to get it. Get the money, right?

FACILITATOR: Okay, yes. Well, tell me about the level of respect you have for Reba now that you got the money. Do you respect her as a person?

ELVIS: No, not really. I just kinda got one on her, you know.

FACILITATOR: Yes, I understand. Now, Reba, tell me about your character in the role play.

REBA: It was awful.

FACILITATOR: What were you thinking?

REBA: I was thinking, "This guy is a jerk."

FACILITATOR: Really? You mean the character Elvis Priestly, of course! Okay, how were you feeling?

REBA: I was angry and irritated. I just wanted him to go away.

FACILITATOR: Yes, I see—What was your sense of closeness with Elvis in the role play?

REBA: Closeness. There really wasn't any. I just felt manipulated.

FACILITATOR: Tell me about your sense of self-respect in the role play. What was that like for Reba?

REBA: I didn't have much. I just thought it was easier to give the money than to argue or fight or whatever.

FACILITATOR: Yes, I see. What sense of respect did you have for Elvis?

REBA: I didn't have any. I didn't really like him or respect him at all.

FACILITATOR: Okay. I see this was a pretty uncomfortable role play then, Reba.

ELVIS: Well, I was doing what I was supposed to do, right?

FACILITATOR: Yes, as Elvis you did a great job of pressuring. And Reba here is just saying how it felt to be in the role of giving in to such pressure. Let's see what the audience observed. Okay, what was the body movement like between these two, audience?

AUDIENCE MEMBER: Elvis kept stepping towards Reba, and Reba kept backing up and turning away. It was like a dance or something.

FACILITATOR: What else, anyone?

AUDIENCE MEMBER: Reba kept wringing her hands and her face was red.

FACILITATOR: What did you observe or imagine about friendship and respect between Elvis and Reba.

AUDIENCE MEMBER: I don't think it was very good. I mean they were like two co-workers or something, but not really friends and they told us the respect was pretty low.

FACILITATOR: Well, what did you in the audience want to see?

AUDIENCE MEMBER: I wanted to see Reba tell him off.

SECOND AUDIENCE MEMBER: I wanted to see Reba say no and stand up for herself.

THIRD AUDIENCE MEMBER: I wanted to see Elvis back off a little bit. I mean it was really clear she didn't want to give him any money.

FACILITATOR: So now you see why we ask you to take a stage name. Sometimes I ask people to play a role that might be less than flattering. So you're giving feedback here to the characters of Elvis and Reba and not really to our volunteers personally, right? Is that clear to everyone? [The group nods in agreement.]

FACILITATOR: Next, after I illustrate a Getting Real response, I want to ask Reba to change her role. Next time, I am going to ask Reba to respond with a "Getting Real" style of communication. Let's review the "When Getting Real" poster on the wall. Can anyone tell me what is different about the Getting Real response?

(The reader should refer at this point to the two Getting Real posters shown in Figures 4.3 and 4.4. One illustrates an adult showing Getting Real communication, and the other describes how Getting Real is done.)

REBA: Well, in this poster, the guy is saying what he really thinks, and he also talks about his real feelings in the situation.

FACILITATOR: Yes, exactly. Sounds easy, doesn't it?

AUDIENCE MEMBER: Well not really, it mostly depends on who you are talking to. I mean it could be really hard, sort of risky and embarrassing, maybe.

FACILITATOR: Yes, I can see that. I'd like to point out that Getting Real techniques seem easier for some people than others. Depending on with whom we are using it, the whole situation can become very close and intimate or it can be painful and risky. So, Getting Real may not be an easy response to use in some situations. I want to direct your attention now to the accompanying Getting Real poster. It states that Getting Real involves confidence,

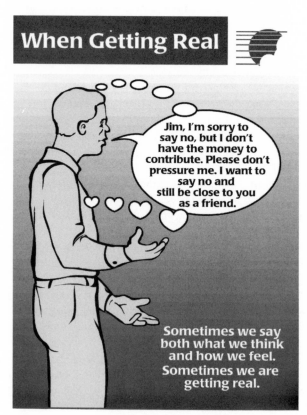

Figure 4.3.

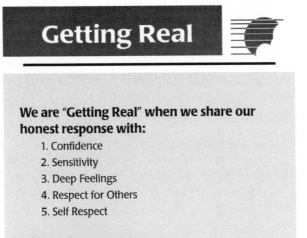

Getting Real

We are "Getting Real" when we share our honest response with:
1. Confidence
2. Sensitivity
3. Deep Feelings
4. Respect for Others
5. Self Respect

It is also important to:
1. Physically show a non-aggressive, firmly-balanced posture
2. Give appropriate eye contact
3. Maintain deep, relaxed breathing and a firm, clear tone of voice

Figure 4.4.

sensitivity, deep feelings, respect for others, and self-respect. Further, it suggests that it is important to show a nonaggressive, balanced posture, using appropriate eye contact. It suggests using deep, relaxed breathing and a firm, clear voice. Wow! That's asking a lot, isn't it?

REBA: Well, it sounds like a lot to remember. I don't know if I can remember all of that and do it up here in front of everyone too.

FACILITATOR: Well, it can be difficult, Reba. May I have your permission to assist you with some direction or prompting as you try?

REBA: Sure, I'll take all the help I can get.

FACILITATOR: Before we even begin, Reba, I want you to stand up with a physical posture that is very balanced and appear confident and proud, but not stiff and uncomfortable. Try to balance your weight on both feet and legs. [Reba adjusts her stance and posture.] Reba, now I want you to breathe in one nice, deep nurturing breath and let it out slowly and fully. See yourself as strong, intelligent, and loving. [Reba breathes in a deep breath and blows it out slowly.] Do you feel a little calmness and strength in this posture, Reba? [Pause—no answer.] I really would like for you to feel good about yourself right now. You know, centered, relaxed, and complete in and of yourself. I want you to feel connected to the ground—fully balanced and relaxed, and connected to yourself—confident and together. And I want you to feel connected to others, too, like everyone matters. Can you get in touch with some of this?

REBA: I think so. I feel a little self-conscious, though.

FACILITATOR: I see. That's understandable up here in front of the group. Yet I want you to see yourself as someone who is very confident. I'll help you too. I'll also ask the group to help you. Is that okay, audience?

SEVERAL AUDIENCE MEMBERS: Yes.

        Go, Reba!

        Go, girl!

FACILITATOR: Reba, you're smiling. That's great! We all want you to be confident and proud. Can you feel it a bit more now?

REBA: Yes, yes, I can.

FACILITATOR: Good. Now try to keep it, because in a moment I'm also going to ask Elvis to pressure you again, and yet I want you to stay confident, caring, and honest, even in the face of his pressure.

REBA: Wow, this could be difficult.

FACILITATOR: Yes, I know, that's why I want to help you. I want you to stand up to Elvis's pressure without fighting him or attacking him or putting him down in any way. And I'll step in and help like a director in a play if you need it—Okay?

REBA: Yeah, okay.

FACILITATOR: And remember, Reba, you really are low on cash, and you don't have any money for this. You really want to say no. And you believe it is okay to say no in this role play.

FACILITATOR (turning now to the other role player):   Okay, Elvis, now I still really want you to get her to give in again—just use any verbal pressure tactic that you want, but remember, no physical contact is allowed. Elvis, are you willing to try to pressure this lady, Ms. Reba McIntosh, into donating to your cause?

ELVIS: Sure, no problem.

FACILITATOR: Reba, are you ready?

REBA: I think so.

FACILITATOR: Remember, Reba, breathe, stay confident and caring, okay? Ready, set, go.

ELVIS: Hello, Reba. You sure look great today.

REBA: Why thank you, Elvis.

ELVIS: Reba, I'm chairman of this fund raising drive and I'm hoping you'll donate ten dollars again this year. I think you gave ten last year, didn't you?

REBA: I don't think so. I don't remember.

ELVIS: Well, I think you did, and besides you are a generous lady—rich and beautiful. I just know you'll help me raise money for these truly needy kids. I mean, some of them need medical operations and food and clothing. Man, it's a cruel world, and I just want you to help make it a little bit better for these kids.

REBA: I don't know, I'm a little short of cash. [She speaks hesitantly and starts to shift her weight back and forth from foot to foot, turning away from Elvis.]

FACILITATOR: Okay, cut. Reba, he's really putting it to you, isn't he?

REBA: Yes, he made up new stuff!

FACILITATOR: Yes, I know he's really pressuring you. How does it feel inside when Elvis does that?

REBA: It's terrible. I feel guilty and pressured. It doesn't seem fair.

FACILITATOR: Okay—I want you to stand firm—physically, hold your ground and stay balanced on both feet. Now, tell Elvis that you feel guilty about not being able to help these children right now. Tell him you're feeling pressured unfairly. Please just tell him you are not able to give this year. Can you do that?

REBA: I think so.

FACILITATOR: Okay, now breathe in, try to stay balanced, and get in touch with your honest position of not being able to give without feeling bad about hurting yourself and your own family.

REBA: Okay. I got it.

FACILITATOR: Okay, Elvis, go back to your line about needy kids, operations and all that stuff. Ready, set, go!

ELVIS: Reba, you're such a beautiful lady—and generous. I know last year you gave ten dollars and that really helped these kids. You know, some of them need food and clothes. Some even need serious medical operations. I know I can count on you for at least ten or twenty, right?

REBA: Well, actually, no, Elvis. I'm short on cash and . . .

ELVIS (interrupting):   That's cool. I'll put it in for you now and you can just pay me back later, Reba—I don't mind. It's for a good cause.

REBA: Elvis, no. I mean it. I don't have the money and I can't borrow it from you now, hoping to pay you later. No, I'd like to be able to give, and I do feel guilty about not giving anything, but I just can't.

ELVIS: Sure you can. I don't care—pay me next month.

REBA: Why don't you just get out of my face. You're a real big jerk . . .

FACILITATOR: Cut! Cut! Please stop. What's happening inside, Reba?

REBA: I'm really getting angry. He won't stop badgering me.

FACILITATOR: Yes, I know—that's his role and he's doing a good job of hassling and pressuring you, isn't he?

ELVIS: I'm sorry—I was just . . .

FACILITATOR: Cut—Elvis, you're just playing a role and doing a good job. Reba is experiencing some powerful feelings here, and it is part of her role. This happens in real life to real people, doesn't it? But this is a role play. You're Elvis Priestly—master pressurer. Reba, you said you're angry to me, but you were attacking Elvis and Getting Rude. Let's try telling him you're getting angry and you want him to stop pressuring you. Isn't that what you really want? Ask him to stop pressuring you—

REBA: Yes.

FACILITATOR: So let's try that. Okay?

REBA: Okay.

FACILITATOR: Elvis, pick up with your I don't care—pay me next month line.

ELVIS: Are you sure it's okay?

FACILITATOR: Reba, can we continue the role play?

REBA: Yes, I guess so.

FACILITATOR: Keep breathing, Reba. You have a right to say no and a right to tell him how you really feel. Try to do it without getting rude or attacking him. I think you can do it.

REBA: Okay, I'm ready.

FACILITATOR: Ready, set, go. Elvis?

ELVIS: Hey, that's okay, Reba. I'll jut put it in now and you can pay me back next month—Okay?

REBA: Elvis, I said no, and you keep pressuring me. I feel bad about saying no, but I mean it. Please stop pressuring me. I'm not going to contribute anything right now. I love kids, I care about you, but I just cannot do it. Please stop asking. It really is hurting me enough already to have to say no, okay? Please.

ELVIS: Well, sure, Reba—I'm sorry. I'm just trying to help the kids, you know.

REBA: Fine, Elvis, but I really can't do it, okay?

ELVIS: Okay, okay—I'm sorry I took it so far, okay?

REBA: Okay, and good luck! I hope someone can help you and the kids out—I'm sorry I can't do it this year.

ELVIS: Okay, Reba—I understand. It's all right. [Spontaneous applause erupts from the audience.]

FACILITATOR: Well, that seemed a little different from the first role play, didn't it? Let's process what this was like first for Elvis and Reba, and then for the audience. Elvis, what was this like for you?

ELVIS: Well, I got uncomfortable with pressuring Reba this time. I felt sort of bad about myself, you know?

FACILITATOR: Yes, I could see a real difference. Tell us what you were thinking this time as Reba was responding.

ELVIS: I was thinking that there was no way she was going to give in, and I better lighten up or I was going to lose a friend.

FACILITATOR: Oh, really—I see. How were you feeling inside?

ELVIS: I was feeling kind of guilty and pushy, and I felt bad about pressuring her.

FACILITATOR: What was your sense of closeness or friendship with Reba?

ELVIS: I found myself caring about how she felt. I felt bad at first, and then I quit pushing so hard and I felt better.

FACILITATOR: So, it seemed hard for you to continue the pressure, huh?

ELVIS: Yes.

FACILITATOR: What was your sense of self-respect like this time?

ELVIS: I felt bad about myself until I quit pressuring her. I was real uncomfortable this time until the end.

FACILITATOR: What would you say about your level of respect for Reba?

ELVIS: I respected her a lot. I was disappointed that I couldn't get the donation, but I really respected her and I wanted her to respect me, so I quit pushing so hard.

FACILITATOR: So she refused you, but you respected her more?

ELVIS: Yes.

FACILITATOR: Would you want to keep her as a friend?

ELVIS: Sure.

FACILITATOR: So you liked yourself more and you liked her more, even though she said no?

ELVIS: Sure! But I was frustrated that I didn't get a donation.

FACILITATOR: I see. Let's check this all out with Reba now, okay?

ELVIS: Sure.

FACILITATOR: Reba, what was this like for you?

REBA: I was nervous and a little scared.

FACILITATOR: Sure, there was a lot of pressure.

REBA: Yes, I know. I really had a lot of emotions going on at one time.

FACILITATOR: I could see it, and you told us too! What were you thinking as these feelings emerged?

REBA: I just wanted it to stop, and I wanted to say no without a big hassle.

FACILITATOR: Sure, tell me about all these feelings you had going on.

REBA: Well, let's see. I was nervous and irritated with all the pressure. But I also felt proud when I really just said no. I was surprised when he finally stopped.

FACILITATOR: Why do you suppose he acted differently toward the end?

REBA: I guess he got the picture.

FACILITATOR: Yes, I think you made your situation pretty clear there toward the end.

REBA: Yes, *after* I did it. It was hard to do at first.

FACILITATOR: It looked hard to do, but I really felt good about you when you did it. How was your sense of self-respect?

REBA: I felt bad about saying no, but I was proud that I stood up for myself. I was surprised and relieved when he stopped pressuring me, too.

FACILITATOR: So you had pretty good self-respect?

REBA: Yes.

FACILITATOR: What about your sense of respect for Elvis?

REBA: Well, I respected what he was trying to do—you know, helping kids and all that. And I also respected him when he listened to me and stopped pressuring me.

FACILITATOR: What about closeness or friendship with Elvis?

REBA: Well, in the end I felt closer than the first time, you know, after he stopped pressuring me and said okay.

ELVIS (interrupting):   Me, too.

FACILITATOR: Okay, let's see what the audience has to say—Group?

AUDIENCE MEMBER: Reba was dancing at first, again, but later on she stood still and held her ground. She was powerful. I really thought she came off well.

SECOND AUDIENCE MEMBER: I liked her a lot more this time and Elvis, too, at the end.

THIRD AUDIENCE MEMBER: I think Elvis could have really turned up the heat.

ELVIS: But I really didn't want to.

FACILITATOR: I see, Elvis, but don't some people just keep pressuring and pressuring, no matter what?

ELVIS: Sure, but I didn't like my role anymore. It wasn't nice or realistic to keep badgering her.

FACILITATOR: Okay, group, tell me about your feelings of respect for these two.

AUDIENCE MEMBER: Well, I liked Reba a lot more this time. I respected her a lot more. I really liked it when she said she cared about the kids and Elvis, too, but wasn't going to give money. I thought that made the difference.

FACILITATOR: She seemed pretty powerful but nice, too, didn't you think?

AUDIENCE MEMBER: Yes, but do you think this always works?

FACILITATOR: Let's see, what does the group say to that?

AUDIENCE MEMBER: Sure it works.

FACILITATOR: Always?

SECOND AUDIENCE MEMBER: No.

FACILITATOR: Why not?

SECOND AUDIENCE MEMBER: Because some people are jerks, and they'll keep it up until hell freezes over.

FACILITATOR: Yes, some people do keep going, and going, and going. How would you respond if they just kept up the pressure even after you Got Real?

THIRD AUDIENCE MEMBER: You would just walk away, wouldn't you?

FACILITATOR: I would like to think so at some point. Would that be Getting Real to walk away?

FOURTH AUDIENCE MEMBER: Yes, that's as real as it gets if somebody just keeps hassling you after you tell him straight out.

FACILITATOR: Sometimes it seems like it's either that, or a fight, or endless hassling. Sure, it's okay to walk away from someone who won't listen to you at all. But can you do that when it's your boss . . . ? Well that's another role play for later maybe. Let's show some appreciation for our two role players!" [Our facilitator leads a gentle round of applause. The group joins in applause.] Let's thank the real people behind the characters of Elvis and Reba. [Here the facilitator says their real names.] Thank you! "I'd like to make a few closing remarks. In this training, the authors are not trying to say that Getting Real is always the *best* response. I believe they are asking us to simply examine the differences between Getting Real and all of the other responses. I believe we all have to choose how we want to respond. And Getting Real may not always be the best choice. Each of us must decide what is best for us in any given situation. Yet it seems nice to know how to Get Real when we really want. What do you think?

We have now examined parts of three different exercises from three different CLFC training components: the first drink/first drunk exercise from Developing Positive Parental Influences; the Feelings exercise from Raising Resilient Youth; and a role play from Getting Real. There is no way that words on paper can engage your mind, body, and heart to the degree that face-to-face interaction can. Yet with a little imagination, the reader can gain a sense of the training experience.

The CLFC program engages the whole person in developing new skills and methods of interaction and emotional processing that lead to behavioral change. Writing about these experiences or reading about them does not begin to compete with, replace, or even truly reveal the power of the group interaction and the intrapersonal dynamics that lead to change. It is our hope that the readers have either experienced this elsewhere in their lives or will make arrangements to participate in this exciting process of enhancing their ability to align their thoughts, feelings, and behaviors in order to gain personal power, human connection and intimacy, and an increased sense of positive and wholesome influence with other people in their lives.

In Chapter 5, we will describe how we have found success in gaining the participation of both parents and youth *and* other community organizations in programming that leads to positive changes in behavior at the individual, family, and community levels.

5

The Creating Lasting Family Connections Community Mobilization Strategy

In Chapters 3 and 4 we focused extensively on the parent and youth training component of CLFC. Chapter 3 also emphasized that while we commonly think of the training component as the main component of a program like ours, we should not overlook the significance of community mobilization.

We believe that mobilizing communities to successfully implement prevention programming *and* (as we will detail in this chapter) increasing the community's capacity to assist families and individuals to deal with the family and societal problems they face are critical to the goals of preventionists. We have found, for example, that after we work with communities to implement our programs, these communities typically show increased demand for additional programming. Moreover, they often show an enhanced ability to successfully implement such programs. We view such changes as critical to achieving the goals we discussed in the introduction to this book. We have already stated that no one can write a program that works for everyone universally. Rather, we need to be engaging entire communities to address the needs of families and youth in programs that enhance the connectedness of people at all levels.

In the sections below, we will first discuss why the community is so important; we will then provide more details of our five-stage strategy to mobilize communities; and finally, we will discuss our vision of how communities, through enhanced capacity and infrastructure, can make a significant difference in the lives of youth and their families.

WHY COMMUNITY MATTERS IN PREVENTION

Communities exert direct influence on the lives of youth, as well as indirect influence on youth through schools, families, and other key institutions. Community-level action (or lack of action) powerfully affects children and youth (Brook et al., 1989; Kelly, 1988). Thus, involving communities in strategies designed to ameliorate social problems like school failure, AOD abuse, delinquency, violence, teen pregnancy, and child abuse can make a critical difference in the life of a child. In this chapter, we describe a specific strategy that we have developed to help communities mobilize for substance abuse prevention.

Bonnie Benard, a leading expert on protective factors, suggests that for youth to become resilient, three characteristics must be present in the family, school, and community domains. These characteristics are caring and support, high expectations, and opportunities for meaningful participation (Benard, 1991). Looking specifically at the community domain, Benard traces these three characteristics in turn, pointing out how each one is essential in helping our youth to become competent to solve problems and to have a sense of purpose and status in their worlds.

Basic caring and support is manifested at the community level in terms of the local resources available to families—these include health care, housing, education, and other key services. Conversely, the greatest risk factor in the development of many problem behaviors is poverty, which clearly implies the lack of such resources. Benard goes on to say that lacking a national will to provide opportunities for all children to succeed, it is up to communities to fill this gap. Benard suggests this be done "through the building of social networks that link not only families and schools but agencies and organizations throughout the community with the common purpose of collaborating to address the needs of children and families" (Benard, 1991, pp. 15–16).

Second, the community impacts families and individuals through high expectations. As Benard points out, these are commonly referenced in terms of "cultural norms." Important norms include the value placed on youth, as well as expectations surrounding the use of alcohol. Benard notes that our culture does not stack up very well in terms of the message it sends regarding responsible alcohol use, partly a result of the large sums the alcohol industry spends to promote its products. Benard states that "the message and expectation that speaks the loudest and clearest to youth is not the one explicitly presented in substance abuse prevention programs in the school but the one implicitly communicated through the values and actions of the larger community" (p. 17).

Third, in terms of opportunities for participation, Benard points out that bonding with the community (developing a sense of belonging and attachment) is dependent on having opportunities to participate in the life of the community. It seems clear that participation in the community may have several beneficial effects on the participating youth and others. Allan Cohen (1991) has argued that participation in the community through volunteer activities may also benefit those helping others, especially with respect to substance abuse prevention. For example, Cohen notes that volunteer helpers can achieve gains in self-esteem, a stronger sense of identity, experiences of meaningfulness, a less passive orientation, and many other benefits. Cohen's view of volunteerism and community service as immunization against substance abuse is clearly related to Benard's point about meaningful participation and involvement.

We have dealt with this topic at some length because it helps clarify some of the key reasons that community matters in substance abuse prevention and other prevention efforts. First, there is the matter of connectedness to the community—and specifically, connectedness to a community that supports and strengthens responsible behaviors in youth. As Cohen points out, when adults and youth become more involved with the community in positive, helping ways, these individuals are also developing personal resiliency through that involvement. As Cohen states, "when we propose voluntary service as an alternative to drugs, we anticipate both the substitution of superior experiences, and an indirect impact on personal and social factors that reduce the personal motivation and social context for substance abuse" (Cohen, 1991, p. 10).

COPES's Experience in Including Community as Part of Prevention

In addition to the abundant support found in the literature pointing to the importance of community involvement, COPES's own program experience over 20 years has underscored the importance of developing involvement at multiple levels. Our experience parallels and reinforces the findings from the research that community level interventions can add real power to interventions targeting youth and their families.

We have also found, however, that the concept of "community" may need to be redefined. Both the literature and our experience led us to redefine the community, based not on geographical boundaries but instead on *natural groupings and support systems where people (individuals and families) have common, and/or shared activities and interests, and social interaction.* The next two sections examine our redefinition in terms of the "village" metaphor.

It Takes a Village, but Is It a Village Anymore?

A popular (and overused) African proverb states: "It takes a village to raise a child." This proverb has been used to symbolize the necessity for community members to pull together to work for their children's best interests. However, we have discovered that in many cases the village no longer exists. The metaphor of the village evokes images of members of a geographical area interacting together, socializing, and working toward everyone's best interest. Yet today, many preventionists target geographical areas where such a "village" does not exist.

The social, economic, and technological changes that have occurred since the late 1940s have contributed to a fragmentation of community life, resulting in breaks in the naturally occurring networks and linkages between individuals, families, schools, and other social institutions within communities. This loss is significant for prevention because it was these networks that traditionally provided the social supports and opportunities for participation and involvement (community resiliency) necessary for healthy human development (Coleman, 1987; Comer, 1984).

Therefore, it has become evident that when they implement programs, preventionists can increase their desired outcomes by rebuilding or re-creating these traditional networks and by deepening any existing linkages so as to increase or reestablish "community" and increase connectedness. Emmy Werner drives this point home in the following statement: "The key to effective prevention efforts is reinforcing, within every arena, these natural social bonds . . . between young and old, between siblings, between friends . . . that give meaning to one's life and a reason for commitment and caring. To neglect these bonds is to risk the survival of culture" (Werner & Smith, 1982, p. 82).

In the next section, we begin discussing our strategy for involving communities by showing how we look at and define "community."

Redefining Community

Many preventionists target communities by defining the community in terms of precincts, census tracts, school districts, or neighborhoods. We believe, however, that it is more important to recognize natural groupings and support systems that still exist. It is necessary to discover where people are currently sharing activities and interests and engaging in social interaction as "community." Trying to target prevention programs for youth and families based on geographical proximity (i.e., neighborhoods, precincts, or census tracts) is often not a viable method.

At the root of our approach to community is the idea that it makes sense to link up with people for prevention where community already exists. This idea grew out of extensive program experience indicating that the use of geographical boundaries in defining communities did not ensure shared activities or interests, and that school communities (and programming) often excluded parents and guardians from their efforts. Therefore, our idea of community is based on the functionality of community members and relationship among members. This definition of community also draws on the literature on functional community organizing (Well & Gamble, 1995). Again, we focus on and utilize a strength that already exists at the community level, just as we did at the individual and family levels (see Chapters 2 and 3).

In today's world, functional/relational communities are not restricted to a geographical area. While people in this type of community may not live in proximity, they do share a concern about a common set of issues relating to the mission of their perceived community. The central focus and desired outcome in mobilizing functional communities is action that emphasizes advocacy and provides services, and that changes policies, attitudes, and behaviors in relation to the targeted issues. In our case, the issues are substance abuse prevention and healthy family interaction and support.

THE CLFC COMMUNITY MOBILIZATION STRATEGY

The CLFC community mobilization process is based on the strategy developed by COPES and implemented through the 5-year CLC high-risk youth research demonstration project. The prototype model has been discussed in several professional articles (Johnson, Noe, Collins, Strader, & Bucholtz, in press; Strader, Collins, Noe, & Johnson, 1996).

The CLFC community mobilization strategy involves a five-stage process of: (1) selecting and recruiting sponsoring community organizations, (2) creating community advocate teams to become successful advocates for ATOD prevention, (3) engaging community advocate teams in recruiting members of the community to receive program services, (4) engaging community advocate teams in retaining participants in the program and its evaluation, and (5) enhancing the community's social services capacity by empowering the community to create self-perpetuating program related initiatives.

Figure 5.1 illustrates the CLFC community mobilization strategy. What follows is a description of each stage of this strategy. This description is specific to the CLFC model. Transferring this mobilization strategy to any other prevention program may require modifications.

Stage I: Selecting and Recruiting Sponsoring Community Organizations

Simply stated, the purpose of Stage I is to identify and select sponsoring organizations that are interested in implementing a family-oriented program. Our program experience tells us, however, that in this and the other stages, it is helpful to have a clear plan of action to ensure that the community can be successfully involved.

The CLFC program can be implemented through multiple types of sponsoring institutions that fit into the definition of community we have described (func-

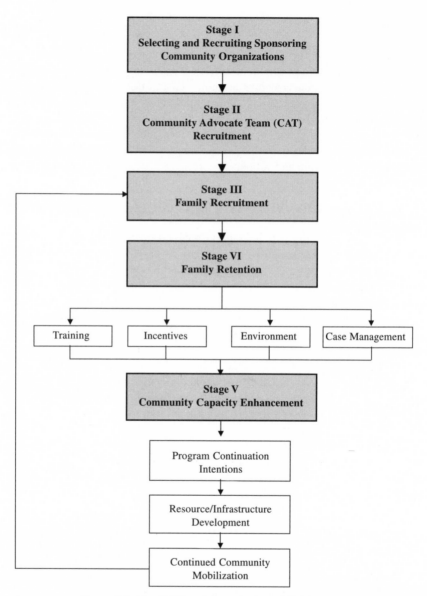

Figure 5.1. The CLFC model community mobilization strategy

tional/relational community), including faith communities, churches with schools, schools, community organizations, agencies, civic groups, recreation centers, or corporations. A sponsoring site can be identified by responding to unsolicited requests from organizations, or program implementers may need to develop marketing/promotions designed to recruit potential sponsoring institutions.

COPES has developed a Creating Lasting Family Connections Site Readiness and Trainer Assessment Survey. It is based on a survey developed by McKelvy, Schneider, and Johnson (1990) for use in the CLC program. Program implementers can send this survey to potential sponsoring organizations, along with a cover letter that will serve as a marketing tool for CLFC. All interested organizations are encouraged to fill out the survey and send it back to the program implementers.

The organizational readiness and trainer assessment consists of four criteria. The first criterion is the number of individuals with targeted characteristics that are accessible within the sponsoring organization's sphere of influence. The second criterion relates to social services or programs recently offered by the sponsoring organization and their relatedness to the CLFC program. The third relates to program offerings by the community organization in terms of whether services were delivered by members of the community organization itself, in cooperation with other organizations, or contracted or referred to external sources (e.g., mental health agencies and self-help groups). The fourth assessment criterion concerns a sponsoring organization's willingness and readiness to implement our program model. To determine readiness, we ask a battery of questions of each site; their responses serve as a "readiness scale" for the prevention effort. These questions measure community priorities, willingness, skills, and resources. That is, they zero in on a community's current level of connectedness.

Once we obtain the survey results, we invite all interested parties that meet our selection criteria to an information meeting where they can learn more about the program and make a commitment to serve as a CLFC site.

In selecting implementation sites, we have identified a cluster of characteristics that enhance the likelihood of success. We have found that success occurs most regularly when we attempt to build from an already existing and successful organization that is willing to act as the foundational platform from which to launch our new program. Other organizational characteristics that we have come to recognize as predictors of success include the following:

- An organization that has at least 100 families as members
- Strong leadership and an established management network
- Leaders who will publicly endorse the program as effective for families
- The existence of regularly scheduled social, recreational, or family-related activities around which recruitment can be planned

It is critical that organizations that are recruited as implementation sites meet the above criteria. Some organizations that appear initially to fulfill the criteria for success on close scrutiny may not do so. For example, a community action group may serve several institutions in its area that do meet the criteria, but the community action group itself does not serve families directly. Even though the community action group has ties with several organizations that have hundreds of members, the community action group itself does not have hundreds of members; therefore, it does not meet the criteria. In this case, the community action group could serve as a liaison and connect program staff to a number of institutions that do meet all of the criteria for a viable site.

Stage II: Community Advocate Team (CAT) Recruitment, Commitment, and Training

While Stage I focuses on acquiring collaboration and program support from a sponsoring community organization, Stage II involves recruiting and training key community leaders from that organization to serve on a CAT. The latter is a group of volunteers recruited and trained to be the outreach arm of the project.

Members of the CAT are recruited using the following strategies. First, a project liaison is selected by the key administrator from the sponsoring organization. The project liaison is responsible for inviting 10 to 12 community leaders (2 or 3 youth and 7 to 9 adults) to an initial CAT overview meeting. The purpose of this meeting is to describe the project, to outline the volunteers' duties, and to recruit at least 8 to 10 voluntary CAT members. Several overview meetings are often required to recruit the targeted number of CAT members who display the qualities essential for program success (i.e., qualities that will also encourage connectedness). These qualities include personal responsibility, strong connections to the community, assertiveness, enthusiasm, promoting of moderate attitudes, openness to new ideas, and good communication skills.

The CAT is a critical feature of our community mobilization strategy for two reasons. First, this group is composed of highly regarded and well-known members within the targeted community. Because of their high visibility and knowledge of other community members, the CAT is able to discern, target, and engage the participation of community members who would likely benefit from our program's services. Second, the CAT provides a familiar face and trusted friend who acts as a liaison between the prevention program provider and community members.

Once the CAT has been recruited, its members are trained so that they are better able to act as successful advocates. Typically, their training requires about four or five sessions, with each session lasting about 2½ hours. During the training, CAT members are provided an accelerated version of the parent and youth training exercises in order to expose them to the training messages, provide them with opportunities to offer feedback on training content, and allow them to offer suggestions, if necessary, for making the training content more culturally relevant for their local community.

We also have found it helpful to provide incentives for CAT participation. For example, CAT members may be offered the following incentives:

- Food and beverages
- Appreciation dinners

- Certificates of appreciation and/or symbolic gifts recognizing status (for example, hats that say "CAT Team Member")
- Child care
- Stipends to help cover transportation or other costs

As the reader can see, many details go into this stage. However, the key point is that Stage II involves recruiting and preparing the CAT. We have learned that having community volunteers so actively involved early on greatly increases community buy-in, thus paving the way for better success at later stages of the strategy.

Stage III: Family Recruitment

During Stage III, the CAT becomes an advocate body for the program's objectives. CAT members are engaged in identifying and recruiting program participants for the CLFC program (and for its evaluation, if needed).

At this stage, the CLFC program providers and the CAT work together to recruit interested youth and families from the community to participate in the CLFC program. This two-pronged recruitment effort helps the CLFC trainers learn more about a given community and its members before being involved in the direct training experience. It also helps maintain a continuous flow of feedback concerning recruitment success.

An important set of events often needs to occur to accomplish the recruitment of the target population. First, the CAT is involved in developing a family recruitment plan in collaboration with the CLFC program training staff. The CLFC program materials include a Prototype Family Recruitment Strategy. This sample recruitment strategy serves as a guide for developing a specific recruitment plan for any community site. However, it is important that the plan be personalized for each community. Because each site has different needs, the success of the recruitment requires CAT input to tailor the recruitment plan to each community and its members' specific needs.

During family recruitment planning meetings, recruitment tasks are identified and CAT members volunteer to carry out the tasks based on a specific time line. Figure 5.2 is an example of a time line used for family recruitment at a hypothetical CLFC community site.

Effective recruitment plans utilize the following activities: recruitment during regular social events, recruitment during rituals and celebrations, endorsements from recognized community leaders, information meetings, advertising in community bulletins, newsletters, and local media, and both telephone and face-to-face contact. It is highly desirable for community members who are targeted for recruitment to experience multiple exposures to the program in a relatively short time period.

Step #	Task/Activity	Date	Person Responsible
1.	Create flyers, brochures, and telephone scripts.	ASAP	TN & WC
2.	Write letter and create invitations to send to families.	ASAP	TN & WC
3.	Call radio stations to ask about public service announcements.	ASAP	WC
4.	Contact newspaper for possible advertisement.	ASAP	CB
5.	Do presentations about program during club member orientation.	Saturdays in Oct.	TW
6.	Meet with basketball teams and schools to inform them about program.	Oct. 1-20	TW
7.	Call local churches to set up meetings to discuss recruitment.	ASAP	WC
8.	Meet with churches.	ASAP	TN & WC
9.	Display flyers and/or posters at local stores.	ASAP	DB
10.	Call Sam to get on the agenda for the Block Watch Meeting.	ASAP	WC
11.	Provide presentation for the Neighborhood Block Watch Committee	Oct. 24	TN or WC
12.	Provide flyers and brochures to the Community Center	ASAP	DB
13.	Mail letters and invitations to families.	Week of Oct. 28	TN, WC & club staff
14.	Phone-a-Thon	Week of Nov. 4	Club staff
15.	Kid's Club	Week of Nov. 4	DB
16.	Canvas the neighborhood with flyers	Nov. 9	TW
17.	Radio PSAs	Week of Nov. 11	WC will coordinate
18.	Advertisements in newspapers	Week of Nov. 11	TN & WC
19.	Send reminder letters to all families on contact sheets.	Week of Nov. 11	TN & WC
20.	Information Night	Nov. 19	All

Figure 5.2. Family Recruitment Planning Worksheet

Without the assistance of the CAT, recruitment of members of a designated target population may be difficult because of the lack of connectedness between the prevention agency and the community members. The creation of a CAT takes full advantage of any existing community bonding, increases this bonding behavior, and draws on this strength to recruit multiple families into the program. Also, the CAT assists in developing and nurturing an array of other resiliency-enhancing activities for families. For example, CAT members help in planning a variety of social events throughout the life of the program that enhance community bonding. In the long run, the community volunteers who make up the CAT help stabilize and sustain community interest and participation in the CLFC program.

Stage IV: Family Retention

The preceding sentence highlights yet another important stage in our community mobilization strategy. Namely, how can we as program staff *stabilize and sustain interest and participation* in the program?

We have noted that family recruitment is critical to the success of our community mobilization strategy. Family retention, that is, keeping the families involved and participating, is likewise of equal value. When the CLFC program targets high-risk youth and their families, the retention stage of the model can be viewed as perhaps the most vital element of the overall strategy. This is so because the effort to retain high-risk youth and their parents in prevention programs is a significant challenge (see Lorion & Ross, 1992). Even among participants who are not high-risk, it is well known that retention efforts can be challenging.

While Stage III involved the CAT's assistance in recruiting participants, it is in the retention stage that CAT members are involved with CLFC trainers in implementing and evaluating a comprehensive program in their community, which requires the ongoing involvement of the CAT. Once again, we have found that careful strategic planning is needed here.

Retention activities are initiated to ensure that participants remain in the program. Unless a sufficient number of participants can be maintained for the duration of the program, it is difficult to bring about the desired behavioral changes among the individual youth, family members, or the community at large.

Four features of the CLFC program have been designed, directly or indirectly, to improve retention: (1) community members' assistance in program implementation and evaluation; (2) enjoyable and effective training experiences for parents and youth; (3) an optional early intervention and case management service for families, if needed; and (4) an optional incentive package. These features can be viewed as a matrix in which each feature works both independent of and in conjunction with the others to create a lasting connection between the program and the targeted community population. Although for discussion purposes and clarity each feature is viewed as a separate entity, retention is most effective when emphasis is placed simultaneously on all program features.

The first feature of the model that aids retention is the involvement of community members (via the CAT) in program implementation and retention activities. After CAT training is completed, CAT members are involved in (1) co-planning the initial strategy to identify the families with high-risk youth, (2) recruiting those families, (3) assisting in scheduling the trainings, (4) refining the strategy for presenting the training in their own community, (5) scheduling evaluation interviews, (6) preparing linkages for successful self-referrals/interventions to service providers, (7) maintaining contact with families throughout the project, and (8) planning and managing the graduation celebration. Thus, the CAT members become energized and engaged in focused behaviors, increasing the community connectedness.

Since parental and family factors are such important influences on youth (see Chapter 2), the CLFC program provides 15 to 20 weeks of 2½-hour sessions that focus exclusively on parents and their high-risk youth. These specific trainings are described briefly in Chapter 3 and in greater detail in Chapter 4.

The use of early intervention and case management services is also viewed as an effective feature to enhance retention. It is important to note that early intervention and case management services, as well as direct incentives, are considered optional features of the CLFC model. Within the CLFC program, the case manager (1) plays the role of trainer or participant-observer during program training sessions, (2) acts as the initial referral source for program participants, (3) initiates contact with all participants who are absent from a training session, and (4) initiates postintervention follow-up services for a predetermined time period.

Case management services greatly enhance the provider's ability to maintain continuous contact with its clientele, which in turn increases the community's desire to continue in the program. Also, by maintaining close relations, participants gain the encouragement and support needed to continue attending the program through to completion, even if personal or family problems arise during the training.

Other incentives also play a key role in the retention stage. Many service agencies have learned through painful experience that despite the strength of a program's core training components, those most in need of services often terminate their involvement prior to program completion (Lorion & Ross, 1992). To address this problem, our mobilization strategy encourages CLFC program providers to offer participants some form(s) of incentive.

One obvious impediment to providing incentives is a tight budget. With this in mind, we have found that a number of innovative incentives are available that can be used with success. Examples of incentives used by the CLFC program have included providing refreshments for participants, providing free daycare through volunteers, making family portraits, providing transportation, having social activities, and giving nominal payments for research interviews (five to ten dollars per interview) when evaluations are conducted. Participants are also invited to add incentives for each other. For example, participants are encouraged to bring their favorite recipes to exchange during breaks in the training, and they are encouraged throughout the program and beyond to support one another's families in multiple ways.

Stage V: Community Capacity Enhancement

Community capacity enhancement is the effective transfer of responsibility for services to the community. This is best achieved both by stimulating community intention to continue programming and by developing community infrastructure and resources. Our experience in implementing CLFC has shown that several things are required to stimulate local community intention to continue program services. Specifically, community leaders need to

- Perceive a need for the services
- Believe in the effectiveness of the services being offered
- Believe that they can successfully continue the services

Regarding the perceived need, since most communities that participate in CLFC have expressed an interest in the program (see the criteria for selection, on p. 69), it is usually clear that they already feel a need for effective prevention services prior to implementation.

Second, the CLFC program has a demonstrated history of achieving positive results among participating families. Therefore, community leaders (CAT members) are able to perceive and promote the services as effective. Then, as local community members engage in the program, either as CAT members or as participants, they too see and feel these benefits firsthand.

Finally, regarding the ability to continue the program, community members gradually come to recognize their own ability to promote the program and to help others gain effective results. This keeps community interest high in making CLFC an ongoing effort in the community. Related to this point, however, is the question of resources. Even though a community may feel a degree of ability to provide services, its success ultimately depends on resources and infrastructure. Therefore, developing infrastructure and resources in the local community is a necessary element if we are to transfer some of the responsibility for continuation of successful prevention programming from a public grant to a self-supporting community function. If we cannot do this broadly and regularly, then substance abuse prevention will remain a government laboratory experiment, viewed by many as another federally funded research project that holds little relevance for communities and families.

Such infrastructure and resource development may take many forms. For example, we have had success in assisting local communities in establishing linkages with outside funding sources that enable them to acquire the resources needed for continuing prevention programming. In some cases CLFC trainers assist community representatives with grant writing and lobbying efforts so that the local community can begin to fund the resources needed to continue the program. In other cases, while the CAT members are involved with the CLFC training staff in their apprenticeship style relationship, CAT members can also be trained to become the management team for the program. Often CAT members are engaged in activities designed to enhance infrastructure, such as institutionalizing the program services within the community's existing service delivery system. Once this management ability is transferred to the local community, it is clear that the community capacity is enhanced, and the community becomes very successfully mobilized.

We believe this transfer of responsibility to the community represents a profoundly important level of program success. In the introduction of this book, we said that it is up to multiple individuals, organizations, and communities to make changes that will have lasting and widespread effects on such issues as youth substance abuse. Thus, our community mobilization strategy has been designed to empower program participants, CAT members, and other community leaders.

In implementing the final stage of this strategy, our prevention service agency plays a relatively passive participant-observer role, so as to shift several responsibilities to the community and away from the agency. The agency may, however, need to continue its relationship with and act on the desires of the community. For instance, if a community wishes to continue the program, in most instances it may need some technical support and assistance. (See Chapter 6 for some details on the technical support and assistance currently available and planned for the future.)

Overall, however, our goal is to encourage communities to develop their own self-perpetuating and self-empowering community initiatives. Our strength is in developing and implementing successful prevention programs; yet communities must build on their own strengths in helping to develop better lives for youth and their families. The reader will see that this chapter has brought us full circle, so that we can now better answer the question of how communities, families, and concerned individuals can actively bring their talents and strengths to bear on issues such as youth substance abuse in a meaningful way that connects the community, its families, and its youth.

6

Questions and Answers about Creating Lasting Family Connections

This chapter addresses the kinds of questions we now receive from those interested in our program. We approached this task by going first to those who have been involved both within and outside of our agency in implementing our programs. We asked them what questions they would still have after reading the information contained in the preceding chapters of this book. Their questions ranged from needing more details on the implementation and evaluation of our program to a more specific concern about how interested organizations and individuals can obtain ongoing information about CLFC.

Question: How do we know that the CLFC program is effective?

CLC, the demonstration program on which CLFC is based, was implemented in urban, rural, and suburban church communities in and around Louisville, Kentucky. The communities served included primarily African-American, as well as primarily Caucasian populations. In CLC, both parents and youth received training, and participating families received early intervention services and follow-up case management.

The evaluation, under the direction of Dr. Knowlton Johnson, of Community Systems Research Division of the Pacific Institute for Research and Evaluation (an independent party), used a true experimental design, in that the youth were randomly assigned to either a program or a comparison group. The evaluation also used three repeated measures over a 1-year period, which allowed the measurement of both short-term and sustained gains. Another strength of the evaluation was that it examined moderating effects of resiliency factors in multiple domains, which "increases the probability of detecting statistically significant results, which facilitates a more accurate understanding of the effects" of the program (Johnson et al., 1996, p. 65).

Some of the main findings included the following. In terms of positive direct effects of the program, there were statistically significant sustained gains by both parents and youth in these areas:

- Use of community services by families with personal/family problems
- Action taken based on the service contact
- Parents' and youths' perceived helpfulness of the action taken

Statistically significant short-term effects of the program on parent and youth resiliency outcomes included the following:

- Increased parents' AOD knowledge and beliefs
- Increased youth involvement in setting AOD use rules

In addition to these statistically significant short-term gains, short-term gains that were close to being significant were noted in the following areas:

- Increased family communication (parent report)
- Increased bonding with mother (youth report)

Besides the program effects described above, the evaluation also included examination of "moderating effects" in which the program was shown to have "produced positive moderating effects on AOD use among youth as a result of conditional relationships with changes in family-level and youth-level resiliency factors targeted by the program" (Johnson et al., 1996, p. 63). For example, a family-level factor that served as a moderator variable for delaying the onset of AOD use was increased program-advocated AOD knowledge and beliefs by parents.

The following were statistically significant moderating effects of family and youth resiliency factors on youth AOD use found through the CLC evaluation:

- Onset of AOD use was delayed among program group youth for 1 year (sustained gain) as parents (1) increased AOD knowledge and beliefs, (2) decreased family conflict (youth report), and (3) increased likelihood of punishing youth for AOD use.
- Use of alcohol was reduced in the short term as parents (1) increased

AOD knowledge and beliefs, (2) decreased their quantity of smoking tobacco products, and (3) decreased their likelihood of punishing youth for misconduct.

For a more detailed discussion of the CLC evaluation findings, the reader is referred to the primary journal article containing the description and results of the evaluation of CLC (the demonstration project from which CLFC was developed). That article appeared in the *Journal of Adolescent Research* (1996). The authors were Knowlton Johnson, Ted Strader, Michael Berbaum, Denise Bryant, Gregory Bucholtz, David Collins, and Tim Noe. In addition to this article, others appeared in the *Journal of Volunteer Administration* (Strader et al., 1997), in *Social Work* (Johnson et al., 1998); and in the *Journal of Community Practice* (Johnson et al., in press).

The reader should note that the program effects found in the CLC evaluation resulted from the implementation of the comprehensive CLC model, which included community mobilization, parent and youth trainings, and early intervention/case management and follow-up services.

Question: If I implement CLFC, how can I measure whether my implementation is successful?

Community Systems Research Institute, Inc. (CSRI) has developed a CLFC evaluation kit to measure the effectiveness of CLFC replications. CSRI developed this kit based on the evaluation design and findings of the CLC demonstration project. The CLFC evaluation kit (Johnson & Young, 1999) is a comprehensive guide for measuring specific outcomes related to CLFC. The kit includes self-administered surveys (based in part on the CLC parent and youth interviews and the CLC youth questionnaire) for both youth and parents, the psychometric properties of the scales in the surveys, survey administration and scoring guidelines, parent consent forms, and contact information for technical assistance on evaluating CLFC.

Question: What are the main differences between CLFC and the earlier CLC?

A key difference is that CLFC, which is the dissemination version of the program, has more flexibility in terms of implementation options. It has a standard implementation option, which uses community advocate teams just as the original CLC did. In addition, we have added a school-based implementation option, in which students (typically sixth to ninth graders) can complete the youth modules either during the course of one school year or by spreading the modules out over three school years. In the school-based implementation option, the parents of the students can be concurrently involved in the parent trainings.

In addition to the school-based option, we have other options that acknowledge that in some situations either the parent trainings or the youth trainings can be implemented without the other. For example, the parent training only option might be used either for a group of parents or as a training for social workers, youth service providers, or other adults who work with youth. Similarly, the youth training only option may be viable in either school settings or other organizational settings where parent participation is not likely.

Figures 6.1 to 6.3 show the Parent Training (Only) option, the Youth Training (Only) option, and the school-based option. The standard option is described in Chapter 3. First, the Parent Training (Only) option can be offered to parents even if their youth do not participate in the youth trainings. Another version of this option is that these trainings can be offered as a training program for social workers, youth service providers, and other caring adults who work with youth. Training these "impactors" can increase our ability to reach youth in a variety of settings.

The Youth (Only) trainings can be offered without the parent trainings. Another variation is that the trainings in the Youth (Only) option can be offered in consecutive years *or* spread over the period of one school year.

Figure 6.3 shows the school-based option. This implementation option is similar to the community-based standard option (see Chapter 3) except that it focuses on sixth to nineth graders. This option can be implemented either with parents and youth *or* with youth only. As with the youth only option, the program can be implemented either over the course of a single school year or over three school years. The actual division of grades in which the modules are implemented depends on the organizational structure of the school system involved.

We have also realized that it is important for agencies and organizations that want to implement science-based prevention programs like ours to have flexibility in the training modules used. For example, an organization or community that wants to implement CLFC may already be successfully using an AOD issues

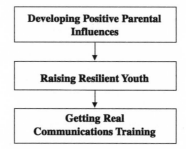

Figure 6.1. Parent Trainings (Only) / training of impactors option.

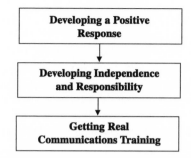

Figure 6.2. Youth Trainings (Only) option.

training. In such cases, it may be beneficial for the community to continue using that ATOD prevention-related issues training, and to combine it with other modules from CLFC in order to establish a more comprehensive prevention program for their community. Combining their existing training modules with ours would not only create a more comprehensive approach, it would reinforce respect for the community investment in programs that they see as their own. This is consistent with our primary belief that it is important in prevention efforts to take advantage of the strengths already present in a community. Any training module or other component used with CLFC must be compatible in its general premises in order to avoid contradictory messages.

Appendix C graphically portrays two ways in which communities might integrate CLFC material into their existing prevention efforts.

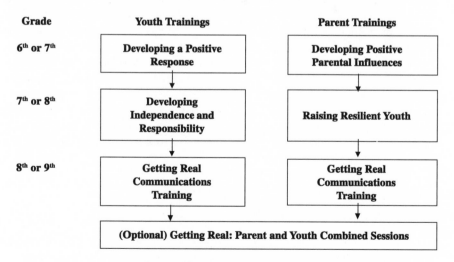

Figure 6.3. School-based option.

Question: How does CLFC achieve involvement of parents?

A significant challenge to the implementation of community-based prevention programs identified by Lorion and Ross (1992) is the difficulty of engaging parents. Yet engaging parents is critical because even though parents often feel inadequate, powerless, or helpless in dealing with a child, research suggests that parental influence is the most powerful factor in prevention (Hazelden Foundation, 1988).

A number of strategies are used to engage parents and other caring adults in the CLFC program. First, in the standard implementation, community advocate teams are recruited and trained to identify and recruit families into the program and to assist in retaining them in the program. These community advocate teams include recognized community leaders who are more likely than outside experts to be able to recruit and retain families successfully.

Second, the parents themselves, once recruited, are actively involved in the parent trainings described in Chapters 3 and 4. Throughout these trainings, the program focuses on the internal motivation that parents possess. We have often noticed that the youth seem to pick up on many of the skills we are teaching more quickly than their parents do, but once both parents and children experience ways in which the training can benefit their families, a synergy develops that can be very powerful.

Third, once families have been recruited into the program, attention must also be given to retention. In fact, Lorion and Ross (1992) cited program retention as another key challenge to community-based prevention programs. Again, the involvement of community advocate teams is critical to addressing this challenge. The team members typically do a number of things to encourage parents and youth to remain in the trainings and other activities. For example, they may call when a family member is absent from a training session to let the participant know that he or she was missed. The participant is often encouraged to return to a warm welcome on the next training date. Finally, participants are gently encouraged to discuss any problems or conflicts they may be experiencing in the training or in their private life that might interfere with their ability to participate. As a result, the case manager is sometimes able to assist with personal problems and help maintain participation.

Question: How does CLFC achieve involvement of youth?

We have successfully engaged youth, as well as parents, in 20 to 25 weeks of training in communication, AOD issues, and other areas of family life. In CLC, the CSAP demonstration project from which we developed CLFC, we achieved the participation even of high-risk youth in this fairly intensive program in a community setting (i.e., where youth participation was not mandatory as it is in some programs, such as school-based prevention programs). This success is a good indication that many youth are motivated to learn.

Again, as with parents, a key to successfully recruiting and retaining youth is to lay the groundwork for the family component by first mobilizing the community. This process was described in detail in Chapter 5. Not surprisingly, many youth seem extremely happy and encouraged to see their parents participate. In some instances, though, children appear uncomfortable or even embarrassed to be seen in their parents' presence. Many children between the target ages of 11 to 17 are experiencing a desire to be perceived as independent of their parents. This is especially true for those from ages 13 to 17. (How many of us parents have noticed the physical distance increase between our children and us as we approach the entrance of Wal-Mart?) Some children, though, also seem to have doubts about their own parents' social acceptability, and this concern may add another level of discomfort to being identified with their parents in public. It is interesting to watch how this dynamic often dissipates after a CLFC facilitator is able to demonstrate a warm acceptance of the parent and the child both separately through individual bonding and collectively, as a family team. Many of these children achieve a new level of acceptance, tolerance, and bonding with their parent by the end of the program.

Question: You have noted that how one defines community is a key to successfully implementing prevention programs. What does this mean for an organization that is interested in implementing CLFC?

We have found through experience that it makes the most sense to link up with people for preventive interventions where "community" of some nature already seems to exist. We also believe that this is true for programs targeting social problems other than substance abuse. "Community" to us means any setting in which people share interests and activities and provide a degree of support for one another. By this definition, a community clearly is not limited to a single geographical entity.

In CLC, we targeted high-risk youth and their families through church communities. In Chapter 5, we described in detail our community mobilization strategy, which was first developed within church communities for the CLC program. Here we would emphasize the importance of flexibility in implementing either the community mobilization component or any of the other program components, including the parent and youth trainings. We found, for example, that each community had varying prevailing attitudes toward such issues as AOD use. By paying attention to these differences and incorporating the input of community leaders into the program presentations, we were able to successfully mobilize a number of communities that were varied in terms of ethnicity, socioeconomic status, and other characteristics.

Variations based on the type of community one is targeting are important as well. For example, in our CLC program, we conducted background research on church communities and found that they share some important characteristics that may set them apart from other types of communities. We found also that church communities tend to be ideal social systems from which to launch preventive programs. There are a number of reasons for this:

- Churches have significant contact with families across their life span.
- Churches often have a number of linkages with human service providers.
- Churches often provide their own social outreach programs.

Different types of communities will have different characteristics that may impact implementation of programs. For example, recreational clubs, such as boys and girls clubs, are very different from churches in terms of parental and youth involvement, and these differences have ramifications for program implementation. Basically, it is important to analyze *how* community is taking place in whatever setting you are involved. It is helpful to ask yourself whether this is a parent-based community, a child-based community, or a family-based community. Churches are often family-based communities; schools are often child-based communities; recreation centers come in both varieties; and corporations are often parent-based communities. Family-based groups are clearly the best places to recruit and retain family participants.

Question: What makes a good trainer for CLFC?

Through COPES's experience of facilitating the curricula described in Chapter 3 (including several earlier versions) with thousands of participants, and from training other trainers to facilitate the curricula, we have learned that specific trainer characteristics increase the likelihood of providing a successful training experience.

The following is a list of characteristics we believe are helpful if one is to be an influential and effective trainer:

1. Outgoing and caring personality
2. Nonjudgmental, tolerant of different opinions
3. Able to handle and accept ambiguity (can see both sides of an issue)
4. Able to hold and model moderate beliefs and attitudes (does not hold or model extreme beliefs and attitudes)
5. Natural helping attitude

6. Has experienced successful group-oriented personal growth opportunities, including counseling, spiritual development, self-help, or related activities
7. Able to recognize, name, and express feelings as they occur

Although anyone who completes our CLFC training of trainers can facilitate the various trainings, trainers who already possess or can quickly learn to display the characteristics listed above will be effective and influential trainers.

In addition, we have found that in order to become a successful trainer, it is important to be able to build meaningful relationships. This takes time, energy, and commitment.

It is helpful to listen to participants and to take them seriously. Once established or strengthened in these relationships, it is helpful to foster responsibility. Responsibility is made up of self-care and care for others. In order to foster this in others, one must demonstrate both self-care and caring for others. Finally, it is important to recognize that extreme attitudes promote extreme behaviors. Moderate attitudes, coupled with a calm approach, take time to develop, but remain effective for long periods of time.

Question: Having discussed characteristics of a good trainer for CLFC, how do you assess trainers' skills and qualities to implement the program? What training do you offer them based on your assessment?

Most people, even experienced preventionists, need some amount of training to engage in the number and qualitative depth of skills required to successfully implement CLFC. In general, those who are inexperienced as prevention trainers are likely to require up to 10 days of training, whereas those who have a good knowledge of prevention and some training experience may require only 5 days of training in order to feel prepared to implement the CLFC program for parents and/or youth.

As we developed CLFC, we saw the need to assess potential trainers' characteristics, experience, attitudes, and values. This assessment was needed to determine whether to conduct a 5- or 10-day training. To address this need, we developed a readiness assessment survey to be administered to all prevention trainers within organizations planning to implement CLFC.

Attitudes and values of trainers are measured by the degree to which they agree or disagree with a number of items around both alcohol and other drug issues and by more general trainer characteristic issues relevant to the CLFC program.

The following statements exemplify the AOD items (preferred responses are shown in parentheses):

- Alcoholics drink alcohol every day. (Strongly disagree)
- It is clearly harmful and dangerous for people to have even one alcoholic drink. (Strongly disagree)
- Regular marijuana use is a harmless and pleasurable practice. (Strongly disagree)

The following are examples of the trainer characteristic and attitude items included in the survey:

- Effective youth workers avoid discussions involving youth feelings of pain, sadness, or anger. (Strongly disagree)
- It is important for children to share in household chores. (Strongly agree)
- Social lies are a good way of protecting people's feelings. (Strongly disagree)
- Every youth group has a few loudmouths and troublemakers who are always going to be problems. (Strongly disagree)

Once an organization's trainers have completed the survey, the instrument is scored by comparing actual responses with desired responses. This score provides a good measure of the kind of training needed by the potential trainers.

Staff members of COPES then discuss these scores with the program manager considering training for his staff or volunteers and negotiate a meaningful training plan by looking at training needs, training budget, schedules, and agency commitment. The training plan is also custom designed based on a dialogue between COPES staff and the organization planning to implement CLFC. Thus, in addition to our 5- and 10-day training plans, we often provide custom trainings for groups that last 3, 4, 6, 8, or 9 days, based on the results of the survey, the agency director's discretion, or (unfortunately) the agency budget.

Question: You discussed what makes a good trainer, but what about community advocate teams? What makes a good team? A good team member?

In our demonstration project, we found that it was desirable for CAT members to have certain characteristics. These include the following:

- Outgoing personality
- Responsibility (for example, is on time for meetings)
- Being well connected to the community
- Possessing leadership qualities
- Assertiveness
- Enthusiasm
- Promoting of moderate attitudes
- Openness to new ideas

The best team size is generally between six and eight active members, depending on the type of setting and the availability of leaders. Also, it is desirable to have both youth and adult members on the CAT. We have found as well that having a variety of personality types on a team is beneficial to group functioning because the different types of leaders complement each other in important ways. The selection and recruitment process is unique in every community.

We are not yet totally confident in our own ability to understand how to get the right CAT members involved. Unfortunately, we often find out the selections were wrong only after recruitment is complete. We slap ourselves on the back and take the credit when the recruitment target is met, but the downside is that we find everyone pointing their fingers at us when recruitment fails. (By failed recruitment, we mean a recruitment drive that results in inadequate numbers of families interested in participating in the program.) To be honest, it is likely that the CAT itself can best perform the postmortem for a failed recruitment drive. This makes sense particularly because they are community members. Sometimes the fault lies with the total apathy within the larger community itself, rather than with any fault of the CAT or CLFC trainers.

Question: In the standard implementation of CLFC, what is the optimum group size for the training for parents? For youth?

In general, we have found that the optimum group size for parents or youth is from 8 to 15, with a maximum desirable size of no more than 25. We based this number on our experience in implementing community, family, and individual youth trainings in a number of different community types, including churches, schools, community organizations, and corporations. The optimum size of 8 to 15 is also consistent with the literature on effective group size (Wheelan & McKeage, 1993; Zander, 1994). For example, Zander (1994) points out that smaller groups foster better involvement and greater harmony, and tend to be more active, cohesive, and productive than larger groups.

Question: What training materials are available for those who want to implement CLFC? What other materials (such as implementation handbooks) do you recommend?

The curriculum materials available include a complete CLFC program package, which contains all five training manuals, a set of 25 participant notebooks for all five trainings, and five poster sets that accompany the training modules. For more information regarding other supporting materials, call our office at (502) 583-6820.

Question: What if my organization wants to write a grant for funding to implement CLFC? Can COPES assist us in this?

Yes, COPES can often assist in grant writing through the provision of supporting materials, letters of support and commitment to provide training, and through review of other grant sections being included in grant narratives. For assistance call or write COPES, Inc. We are also currently developing a question-and-answer center on our Web site. This is likely to become something like a CLFC chat room. While this question-and-answer chat room is not operational at the time of this writing, it is scheduled to be operational by the date of publication. Our Web site is located at COPES.org.

Question: What is the average cost for implementing CLFC?

If the organization already has skilled and experienced staff (see question above), then the only cost would be the cost of the curriculum materials (from $1500 to $2000). However, an organization would typically need to budget at least $750 per week of training needed per trainee, plus travel costs to a training site near them. If an organization or a group of organizations has several people who need trainings, the cost can be reduced. Please call COPES, Inc. to examine a variety of training options.

Question: What generally is involved in the CLFC implementation training?

Typically, the potential trainers would be taken through an abridged version of all of the CLFC training modules to gain an understanding of what it means to be a participant in these trainings. Next, potential trainers would be provided an in-depth training on each of the modules. In this portion of the training, they would be given tips on how best to engage participants in the various modules. Finally, a component of the training of trainers consists of "mock" training exercises, in which participants act as trainers and are subsequently given feedback from the group.

Question: Does completion of the CLFC implementation training qualify a trainer to train others who are interested in implementing the CLFC program in other communities?

The CLFC implementation training is designed to provide the skills necessary for implementing CLFC with youth and families in one's community. It is not designed to empower people to train others to implement CLFC. That requires both successful implementation of our program and successful completion of our CLFC Master Trainers course. Certified Master Trainers are eligible to receive compensation (travel, per diem, and training fees) from COPES, Inc. for conducting certified implementation trainings.

Question: Your CLFC program appears to go pretty deep. Is this therapy?

Yes, our program goes into each topical area with a fair degree of depth, but it is not the same as therapy. No counseling is involved. The program can and does have a therapeutic effect on some individuals and families. The program is clearly an educational and skill-building program designed to be provided in a group setting. The skills that are taught and practiced in the curriculum are very positive and nurturing practices that certainly impact the individual who learns and uses them. It is not at all surprising that these improvements in one family member (parent) would also impact others in the family.

Question: Do you think most grass-roots facilitators are qualified to become CLFC trainers and take on such a deep and powerful role?

This sounds like two separate but related questions. First, is it appropriate for "regular" people to lead or facilitate this type of family program? And second, can "regular" people really facilitate this program?

Yes, we believe it is very appropriate for "regular" people to make a conscientious effort to assist others who have children to raise them successfully. And we believe that many adults outside the nuclear family can and should provide a positive influence on other community members' children especially when the children's parents need and request assistance. Raising children is a deep and powerful responsibility that in most cultures has been shared with others outside of the immediate family for centuries. It's virtually unavoidable anyway. Simply stated, we believe that those of us who are willing to help others who want and/or need our assistance can learn to improve our methods as we assist them.

Further, we believe that "regular" people are essentially the best suited to become CLFC trainers. By "regular" people we mean that people are not required to have an advanced degree in psychology, counseling, education, or sociology to become a CLFC trainer. On the other hand, to possess such a degree would not be a disadvantage either. The skills promoted in the CLFC program are human skills. We believe anyone who wants to improve his or her skills and is willing to assist others with improving skills can do so. We provide a skill-building training for adults who are interested in implementing this program with others. Anyone who has access to our materials and is comfortable enough with the program to implement it with others can justifiably do so. Many people gain great confidence in their CLFC facilitation skills as a result of receiving our implementation training.

Question: Your training seems very sophisticated. How well does it work with uneducated or economically disadvantaged families?

Our training is comprehensive and systematic so it might be fair to call it sophisticated. We certainly understand your question, too. When we first designed the research model, CLC, we intended it for use with high-risk youth and families. We were concerned that it might be overwhelming for some of them, or even turn them off. Yet in our implementation of the program, we did not experience any major negative reactions to its sophistication. There were three reasons that we think we were able to reduce this possible tension. First, people were told to use the workbooks only if they preferred to do so. We told them we recognized that some people hate or struggle to read, while others enjoy it. We showed respect for either choice or preference. The training is designed to be primarily interactive and experiential, and they were assured that participants would receive the majority of benefits from our program simply by showing up for the trainings and participating. We were not uptight about people choosing not to read or even accept the participant notebooks or handouts.

Second, the program is designed to support the parent as the decision-maker in the family. We took care to ensure that the program does not preach, judge, or stigmatize in any way people who attend. No one is forcing attendance, homework, or even ideas onto anyone else. We worked hard to develop a local CAT to help us create the right atmosphere around the program, and this helped us put people at ease.

Finally, because we were the facilitators in this research study, we already had experience working with families such as these and we were thus very comfortable working with them. The facilitator is the centerpiece of this training once the families have been recruited by the CAT. We really believe that if the facilitator is comfortable with his or her role, is familiar with the materials, and is accepting of the participants, then everyone is likely to have a very positive and affirming experience.

We would also like to acknowledge that we have had times when people signed up for the program who apparently had no genuine intention of becoming truly involved. This occurred in the program with the CAT. You will find people (of all socioeconomic and educational levels) who appear to be reluctant to say no—even to one of their own community members. They say yes, sign up, and then never show up. This is unfortunate because they would especially benefit from our Getting Real training, which assists people who have difficulty saying no.

Question: How do you make your training culturally relevant for minority populations?

We make a serious attempt to design our program to draw on the "human experience" rather than to focus on any individual experience. Regardless, we recognize that all of us as authors or curriculum developers are still limited by our individual and cultural experiences, even though we may have broad cultural experience. We engineered cultural input from the target population by creating the CAT component as part of our community mobilization design. The CAT is expected to teach, mentor, or otherwise instruct the program facilitators in gaining an understanding of the local cultural issues and to provide a two-way bridge of understanding and acceptance between the participant population and the facilitator(s). This unique design feature has proved to be indispensable because it is so effective in overcoming cultural, social, and related differences between (and among) facilitators and participants.

Question: Violence is a big issue right now. How does your program target violence prevention?

Our CLFC program includes five training modules. Two of these modules have a direct bearing on violence-related factors, and all five send a comprehensive message of acceptance, inclusion, and respect for others. We believe that people who experience large amounts of acceptance, inclusion, and respect likewise experience an increased sense of connection with others and are therefore much less likely to become involved in violent behaviors. The two training components that deal very directly with violence reduction are Raising Resilient Youth and Getting Real. The Raising Resilient Youth training encourages parents to avoid physical or corporal punishment as a primary means of influencing their children's behavior. Children who typically experience regular physical punishment or abuse are at a greater than normal risk of engaging in aggressive and violent behavior. In the Getting Real curriculum, both youth and parents are encouraged to role-play a variety of pressure situations that might trigger a powerful emotional reaction. Participants are taught the Getting Real response, which incorporates respect, confidence, friendship (if possible), and honesty. These responses move the situation away from conflict and the likelihood of violence. Further, Getting Real teaches both youth and adults how to exit an escalating conflict where resolution appears unlikely.

Unfortunately, we did not include any violence measures in our original research design. Therefore, we currently lack scientific evidence on which to claim violence reduction as an outcome. We are looking for an opportunity to examine violence-related outcomes in our next study.

Question: What are some common problems people encounter when using your program?

There are several pitfalls that we have encountered when implementing this program and that others have experienced too. The biggest potential problem is low recruitment and/or high attrition. It is hard to recruit families for almost any type of event, and this is especially true for an 18- to 20-week program involving both parents and youth.

The list of reasons why our own recruitment efforts have suffered in the past is already long and continuing to grow. The most common problem is poor planning and overly optimistic expectations at the beginning of an implementation. We now often spend up to 6 months of fairly intensive time and energy in the community mobilization phase. Identifying the right community and the right community leaders to support a recruitment drive is critical. Next, we've learned to pay attention to subtle but nevertheless clear indicators that recruitment is not going to go well in a given setting. If community advocate teams are hard to develop, then recruitment is likely to be impossible. Sometimes we target communities not yet ready to receive our message. Discretion may help us avoid wasting a lot of time and effort attempting a recruitment drive when indications are that a community is not ready to support it. It is important to avoid the trap of assuming that because a community is experiencing a drug problem, the community members will really want the program. Sometimes the worse the problem appears in an area, the harder it will be to gain widespread support for a prevention program.

Next, we have sent inappropriately skilled or trained staff out to recruit in communities to which they are poorly suited. While race, gender, and age immediately come to mind, our most serious errors have occurred when our own representatives have not had faith, confidence, or real respect for community members or leaders they were asked to engage. Prevention staff promoting the program must truly believe in themselves, the materials, and target population members' ability to ultimately care for themselves and their children.

Another real problem occurs when a community group is concerned about the substance abuse problem and really wants to push for the program in their community. We have encountered this problem in a variety of forms over the years. The problem often first shows up as an apparent minor variance in philosophy between community leaders and our program model. Typically these leaders have a subtle anger, resentment, or judgment hidden beneath the surface in their motivation to "help" the community. Notice how above we said that they want to "push" for the program. No one, however, really wants to be pushed into a program. Gentle but clear confrontation whenever even small hints of this type of attitude are expressed by community leaders or CAT members helps to avoid problems of this type. We've come to the conclusion that if this type of push/pull mentality continues after we've confronted it early and often, it may be better to move our recruitment efforts elsewhere.

Finally, we've encountered some problems with extremely difficult participants. It usually isn't someone who is consciously trying to cause a problem. Most often it is either someone in a crisis who simply dominates the group discussions and overwhelms the trainer and group with personal needs and questions, or it is someone who is seriously challenged intellectually or who is emotionally disturbed and he or she is impossible to manage in a group setting. These individuals usually need a more focused effort and benefit from receiving a referral to a more appropriate individual counseling setting. Other participants can be "run off" if the trainer does not intervene early enough and yet the converse is also an issue. Trainers are wise to remain somewhat accepting of individuals who occasionally exhibit mildly inappropriate behavior. We have found it helpful to acknowledge these behaviors as inappropriate while supporting and accepting the individual involved. If this approach is not adequate to cause some improvement in the participant's behavior, a private meeting may be required to make the trainer's expectations very explicit.

Any individuals or groups experiencing any implementation challenges in using our curricula are encouraged to call our office for suggestions and consultation.

Question: Okay, I'm convinced your program is worth purchasing. How can I convince my boss or the other community leaders to purchase and implement your program?

We do not have any magic response to this question. We do, though, have a wealth of experience in helping people who share this need to gain the necessary support of others to get the program started in their organizations. We can offer without charge some very attractive promotional materials that you can use to help educate and persuade the decision-makers in your community. In addition, we are often available for a limited amount of free telephone consultation to assist you in this effort. Feel free to call our primary author, Ted N. Strader, at (502) 583-6820 for assistance in these matters.

Conclusion

We wrote in the introduction that we are not the first generation of adults to experience pain, frustration, and even fear in dealing with our youth. It is important that parents, teachers, and all others who interact with youth also recognize and validate these feelings as they arise in themselves and in others. Equally important is to recognize that our youth embody all hope and aspirations we share for the future of humanity. They are worth the considerable effort, expense, and personal investment we are required to make. Our own generation's historical worth and value may be, and probably will be, measured by the extent to which we succeed or fail to socialize our youth. We are inextricably connected to them for better or worse.

We have created this program and focused virtually all of our prior efforts in order to improve the quality of our own lives with a hope that what we do through this program may impact in a positive and meaningful way others who follow. How did we do this? We did it with science. Science asks us to study preceding generations, to examine prior successes and failures. Thus, Chapter 1 included a brief outline of the history of substance abuse prevention in the United States. We learned everything that we know from an integrated application of some methods that showed promise that some brave pioneers had implemented earlier. Our study also helped us avoid the unproductive approaches that others had tried and found unworthy in the past.

Next we provided a description of our own prevention approach embodied in the CLFC model and shared the results of the "outside" evaluation conducted on our research demonstration project. Others in the field—most notably CSAP and the International Youth Foundation—found our program worthy of dissemination and replication based on these results. We continue to perceive ourselves and the entire field of prevention (and our nation as a society), however, as less than adequately prepared to accomplish the level of results necessary. Thus, we are far from ready to begin the celebration. While our results may appear impressive to others and we are encouraged by that, we are not very well satisfied that this represents the full extent of our potential influence. We liken our experience to that of a young man at a county fair. He steps up to the giant hammer, hoping to bring it down with such force as to drive the small metal weight up the entire shaft in order to ring the bell at the top. He swings the hammer with all his might and it comes down with only enough force to raise the metal weight to the height labeled "weakling." Yes, he moved the weight up the shaft in the right direction, but only enough to show a fairly clear lack of strength, leverage, or technique. Yes, the moderating effects of our program have demonstrated a delay in the onset of substance use for some youth, and reduced current use for others. But we certainly have not created a universal vaccine.

So after describing the historical context, general theory, and specific design and results of our program, we tried to illustrate the art and craft of implementation by including sample exercises from our training components that would give the reader a deeper and more concrete sense of how it works. We fully recognize the limitations in attempting to describe in writing that which will play out uniquely in every setting. We hope the reader will be able to gain enough of the flavor from these brief samples to take an even larger taste by examining our full curriculum materials and training experience—and perhaps even by implementing our entire program. Our ultimate desire is that other professionals in the field of prevention will use our efforts in this arena as a springboard to even greater results. We believe our future as a society and even as a race depends on this effort.

Appendixes

A

Resiliency Factors by Domains and CLFC Components

Resiliency factor	CLFC component targeting the factor
Community domain	
• Recruitment and retention of families	• All community mobilization activities
• Empowerment by community advocate teams	
• Participation in project activities	
School domain	
• Recruitment and retention of families	• All school community mobilization activities
• Empowerment by community advocate teams	
• Participation in project activities	
• School climate	
Family domain	
• Appropriate ATOD knowledge and beliefs	• Developing Positive Parental Influences
	• Developing Independence and Responsibility
• Parents' situational use of ATOD	• Developing Positive Parental Influences
• Frequency of family meetings	• Raising Resilient Youth
• Bonding with youth (youth report)	• All parent and youth trainings
• Communication with youth	• Getting Real
	• Raising Resilient Youth
• Involvement of youth in setting non-ATOD rules	• Raising Resilient Youth
• Involvement of youth in setting ATOD rules	• All parent and youth trainings
• Help-seeking for family problems	• All parent and youth modules
• Positive consequences for youth following important family rules	• Raising Resilient Youth
	• Developing Independence and Responsibility
	• Developing Positive Parental Influences

(continued)

99

(continued)

Resiliency factor	CLFC component targeting the factor
• Negative consequences for youth breaking important family rules	• Raising Resilient Youth • Developing Independence and Responsibility • Developing Positive Parental Influences
• Family stability and cohesiveness	• All parent and youth modules
• Reduced family conflict	• All parent and youth modules
• Family recreation and community activities	• All parent and youth modules
Individual domain	
• Appropriate ATOD knowledge and beliefs	• Developing a Positive Response
• Attitudes unfavorable to ATOD use	• Developing a Positive Response
• Refusal skills	• Getting Real
• Bonding with mother	• All youth and parent modules
• Bonding with father	• All youth and parent modules
• Honest and open communication	• Getting Real
• Participation in family rule setting (non-ATOD)	• Developing Independence and Responsibility • Developing Positive Parental Influences
• Participation in family rule-setting (ATOD)	• Developing Independence and Responsibility • Developing Positive Parental Influences
• Bonding with community	• All youth and parent modules
• Social skills	• Getting Real

The CLFC Program
Logic Model

Logic models, according to the National Institute on Drug Abuse (1997a), are "graphic summaries of the essential elements of strategic plans." This same source also says that logic models usually specify the specific prevention activities that will be implemented, the anticipated immediate or short-term effects (objectives) of these activities, and the anticipated long-term outcomes or goals achieved by participants (National Institute on Drug Abuse, 1997a, p. 88).

First, we briefly describe how we developed our logic model. Then we briefly illustrate how it can be used to help evaluators, prevention specialists, and community members understand the linkages between long-term objectives, resiliency factors, measurable objectives, and program components.

Table 1 outlines the logic model used to design the CLFC project. The first step in developing the logic model was to identify the specific resiliency factors in each of the domains (community, family, school, and individual youth) that are correlated with youth ATOD use. These resiliency factors were identified with input from community representatives, research conducted in the targeted areas, and relevant literature. The second column in Table 1 shows the resiliency factors targeted. For example, under the heading of "Youth" in that column, "youths' unfavorable attitudes toward ATOD use" is one of the resiliency factors listed. As stated earlier, the importance of youth attitudes toward ATOD use has been clearly established in the prevention literature.

Note that in Table 1, the long-term objectives are both delaying onset of AOD use and reducing frequency of AOD use.

The second step in developing the logic model was to establish the specific measurable intermediate objectives the program would target based on the identified resiliency factors. It was important that the objectives be directly linked to the specific resiliency factors. Again, using the example of youth attitudes toward ATOD use, the specific measurable objective was to increase youths' unfavorable attitudes toward ATOD use.

The third step in developing the logic model was to design the interventions to address these specific resiliency factors and, in turn, meet the proposed objectives. The interventions chosen for the CLC program were designed to provide five broad approaches to prevention/resiliency building: community mobilization; individual and family skill building; raising awareness, motivating, and educating; providing alternative activities and encouraging the incorporation of these activities into the daily lives of targeted families; and providing advocacy and modeling it for the community so that ongoing advocacy for prevention might continue after the program.

To demonstrate how the logic model functions in linking program components to resiliency factors and measurable objectives, consider the resiliency factor of bonding within the family. As we described earlier in this book, considerable empirical evidence exists to support that bonding in the family is an important resiliency factor in terms of adolescent drug use. In other words, stronger family bonding tends to be associated with less adolescent drug abuse.

As we developed our logic model, we built in "youth bonding with parents" as a targeted resiliency factor (see second column), and we stated a measurable objective as an "increase in bonding with parents" (see third column). In our original research, this objective was stated as "there will be a statistically significant increase in family bonding."

Having stated a measurable objective in terms of change in family bonding, the next step is to make sure that there are elements within program components that will address this resiliency factor. In terms of our program model, all three of the parent components and all three of the youth components placed some emphasis on youth bonding with parents. In the parent trainings, for example, the Raising Resilient Youth training module increases bonding as it teaches and encourages parents to include their children's participation in the setting of expectations and consequences for a variety of behaviors. The Getting Real training for parents, for youth, and for both parents and youth combined also enhances bonding through a better understanding (and practice) of communication styles that lead to mutual awareness and self-respect.

Some resiliency factors are more closely associated with specific components. For example, we would expect that "youths' unfavorable attitudes toward ATOD use" would be increased especially through the Developing a Positive Response module, since this is the module within CLFC designed specifically around ATOD issues for youth.

Table 1. Logic Model for CLFC

Long-term objectives	Resiliency factors targeted	Intermediate objectives	Intervention components
Youth	*Community:*	*Community*	*Community*
• Delay onset of alcohol and other drug use	• Community engagement	• Successfully engage communities to implement CLFC	• Community Mobilization Component (CAT recruitment and development; CAT training)
• Reduce frequency of alcohol and other drug use	*Family* • Parents' situational use of ATOD	• Communities successfully recruit and retain families	*Parent*
	• Family meetings	• Communities sustain prevention efforts	*Three modules*
	• Help-seeking for family problems	*Family*	• Developing Positive Parental Influences
	• Positive communication with youth	• Increase appropriate situational use of ATOD	• Raising Resilient Youth
		• Increase frequency of family meetings	• Getting Real Communication Training
	• Youth involvement in setting family rules	• Increase help-seeking for family problems	*Youth*
		• Increase positive communication with youth	*Three modules*
	• Positive consequences for youth following important family rules	• Increase youth involvement in setting family rules	• Developing a Positive Response
		• Increase positive consequences for youth following important family rules	• Developing Independence and Responsibility
	• Negative consequences for youth breaking important family rules		• Getting Real Communication Training
		• Increase negative consequences for youth breaking important family rules	*School*
	• Family stability and cohesiveness		• Any or all youth and/or parent modules (listed above) implemented in a school setting
	Youth:	• Increased family stability and cohesiveness	
	• Youths' Getting Real communication	*Youth*	
	• Youths' unfavorable attitudes toward ATOD use	• Increase Getting Real communication	
		• Increase unfavorable attitudes toward ATOD use	
	• Help-seeking	• Increase help-seeking	
	• Youth bonding with parents	• Increase bonding with parents	
	• Youth bonding with community	• Increase bonding with community	
	• Youth bonding with school	• Increase bonding with school	
	• Youth school attendance	• Improved school attendance	
	School	*School*	
	• School climate	• Improved school climate	

C

Integrating CLFC Materials into Community Prevention Efforts

In Chapter 6, we stated the importance of agencies and organizations enjoying a certain degree of flexibility in the CLFC training modules they implement. The following figures illustrate two common ways in which agencies or organizations might integrate CLFC components with their own existing prevention approaches. In Figure 6, a community which already has its own youth alcohol and other drug issues training (called "Cool Cats Don't Use") has integrated its youth training module into the CLFC youth modules. In this example, "Cool Cats Don't Use" replaces the CLFC Developing a Positive Response module.

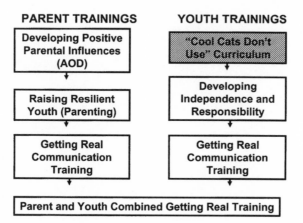

Figure C.1. Sample Integration #1.

In Figure 7, a community, "Cat City," with a fairly sophisticated (multiple domain) prevention effort already in place, has integrated the CLFC parent and youth Getting Real training modules into its effort. When integrating components from separate prevention programs, care should be taken to ensure that the appropriate risk and protective factors are targeted by the specific components selected for implementation.

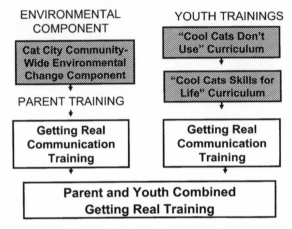

Figure C.2. Sample Integration #2.

References

Ahmed, S. W., Bush, P. J., Davidson, F. R., & Iannotti, R. J. (1984). *Predicting children's use and intentions to use abusable substances.* Paper presented at the Annual Meeting of the American Public Health Association, Anaheim, CA.

Anderson, A. R., & Henry, C. S. (1994). Family system characteristics and parental behaviors as predictors of adolescent substance use. *Adolescence, 29*(114), 405–420.

Atkin, C., Hocking, J., & Block, M. (1984). Teenage drinking: Does advertising make a difference? *Journal of Communication, 34,* 157–167.

Bandura, A. (1986). *Social foundations of thought and action: A social cognitive theory.* Englewood Cliffs, NJ: Prentice-Hall.

Barnes, G. M. (1990). Impact of the family on adolescent drinking patterns. In R. L. Collins, K. E. Leonard, & J. S. Searles (Eds.), *Alcohol and the family: Research and clinical perspectives* (pp. 137–162). New York: Guilford.

Barnes, G. M., & Welte, J. W. (1986). Patterns and predictors of alcohol use among 7th–12th grade students in New York state. *Journal of Studies on Alcohol, 47,* 53–62.

Beck, J. (1998). 100 years of "just say no" versus "just say know": Reevaluating drug education goals for the coming century. *Evaluation Review, 22*(1), 15–45.

Benard, B. (1991). *Fostering resiliency in kids: Protective factors in the family, school, and community.* Portland, OR: Northwest Regional Educational Laboratory.

Brook, J., Nomura, C., & Cohen, P. (1989). A network of influences on adolescent drug involvement: Neighborhood, school, peer, and family. *Genetic, Social and General Psychology Monographs, 115*(1), 303–321.

Brook, J. S., Brook, D. W., Gordon, A. S., Whiteman, M., & Cohen, P. (1990). The psychosocial etiology of adolescent drug use: A family interactional approach. *Genetic, Social and General Psychology Monograph, 116,* 111–267.

Brook, J. S., Lukoff, I. F., & Whiteman, M. (1980). Initiation into adolescent marijuana use. *Journal of Genetic Psychology, 137,* 133–142.

Brook, J. S., Whiteman, M., Gordon, A. S., & Brook, D. W. (1988). The role of older brothers in younger brothers' drug use viewed in the context of parent and peer influences. *Journal of Genetic Psychology, 151,* 59–75.

Casey, E. (1979). A history of drug use and drug users in the United States. In *Drugs in Perspective: Participant manual* (NIDA), 79–132.

Center for Substance Abuse Prevention (1997). *Guidelines and benchmarks for prevention programming.* Rockville, MD: Author.

Cohen, A.Y. (1991). *Volunteers in prevention.* Pacific Institute for Research and Evaluation. Bethesda, MD: Potomac Press.

Coleman, J. (1987). Families and school. *Educational Researcher, 16*(6), 32–38.

Comer, J. (1984). Home-school relationships as they affect the academic *success* of children. *Education and Urban Society, 16*(3), 323–337.

COPES (1998a). *Creating Lasting Family Connections, Developing a positive response manual.* Louisville, KY: COPES, Inc.

COPES (1998b). *Creating Lasting Family Connections, Developing independence and responsibility manual.* Louisville, KY: COPES, Inc.

COPES (1998c). *Creating Lasting Family Connections, Developing positive parental influences manual.* Louisville, KY: COPES, Inc.

COPES (1998d). *Creating Lasting Family Connections, Getting real manual.* Louisville, KY: COPES, Inc.

COPES (1998e). *Creating Lasting Family Connections, Raising resilient youth manual.* Louisville, KY: COPES, Inc.

Dishion, T. J., Kavanaugh, K., & Kiesner, J. (1998). Prevention of early adolescent substance abuse among high-risk youth: A multiple gating approach to parent intervention. In R. S. Ashery, E. B. Robertson, & K. L. Kumpfer (Eds.), *Drug abuse prevention through family interventions* (NIDA Research Monograph 177). Rockville, MD: National Institute on Drug Abuse, 208–228.

Feldman, R., Stiffman, A., & Jung, K. (Eds.). (1987). *Children at risk: In the web of parental mental illness.* New Brunswick, NJ: Rutgers University Press.

Florin, P., & Wandersman, A. (1990). An introduction to citizen participation, voluntary organizations and community development: Insights for empowerment through research. *American Journal of Community Psychology, 18,* 41–54.

Garmezy, N. (1985). Stress-resistant children: The search for protective factors. In J.E. Stevenson (Ed.), *Recent research in developmental psychopathology. Journal of Child Psychology and Psychiatry, 4,* 213–233.

Goodstadt, M. S. (1986). School-based drug education in North America: What is wrong? What can be done? *Journal of School Health, 56*(7), 278–281.

Greenblatt, J. C. (1998). Adolescent self-reported behaviors and their association with marijuana use. In *Analyses of substance abuse and treatment need issues.* Rockville, MD: SAMHSA, 89–109.

Gurian, A., & Formanek, R. (1983). *The socially competent child: A parents' guide to social development—From infancy to early adolescence.* Boston: Houghton Mifflin.

Hansen, W. B., Graham, J. W., Sobel, J. L., Shelton, D. R., Flay, B. R., & Johnson, C. A. (1987). The consistency of peer and parent influences on tobacco, alcohol, and marijuana use among young adolescents. *Journal of Behavioral Medicine, 10,* 559–579.

Hawkins, J. D., Catalano, R. F., & Miller, J. Y. (1992). Risk and protective factors for alcohol and other drug problems in adolescence and early adulthood: Implications for substance abuse prevention. *Psychological Bulletin, 112,* 64–105.

Hazelden Foundation (1988). *It's time to talk.* Minneapolis, MN: Author.

Jaffee, D. (1974). Drug laws: Perceptions of illegal drug users. *Drug Forum, 3*(4), 321–329.

Johnson, C. A., & Solis, J. (1983). Comprehensive community programs for drug abuse prevention: Implications of the community heart disease prevention programs for future research. *National Institute on Drug Abuse Monograph Series, 47,* 76–114.

Johnson, K., Bryant, D., Collins, D. A., Noe, T. D., Strader, T. N., & Berbaum, M. (1998). Preventing and reducing alcohol and other drug use among high-risk youth by increasing family resilience. *Social Work, 43*(4), 289–384.

Johnson, K., Noe, T., Collins, D., Strader, T., & Bucholtz, G. (in press). Mobilizing church communities to prevent alcohol and other drug abuse: A model strategy and its evaluation. *Journal of Community Practice.*

Johnson, K., Strader, T., Berbaum, M., Bryant, D., Bucholtz, G., Collins, D., & Noe, T. (1996). Reducing alcohol and other drug use by strengthening community, family, and youth resiliency: An evaluation of the Creating Lasting Connections program. *Journal of Adolescent Research, 11*(1), 36–67.

Johnson, K., & Young, L. (1999). *The Creating Lasting Family Connections Program Evaluation Kit.* Louisville, KY: Resilient Futures Network.

Johnston, L. D., O'Malley, P. M., & Bachman, J. G. (1999). *National survey results on drug use from the Monitoring the Future study, 1975–1998.* Rockville, MD: National Institute on Drug Abuse.

Kaftarian, S. J., & Hansen, W. B. (1994). Improving methodologies for the evaluation of community-based substance abuse prevention programs [CSAP special issue]. *Journal of Community Psychology Monograph Series*, 3–5.

Kandel, D. B., Kessler, R. C., & Margulies, R. S. (1978). Antecedents of adolescent initiation into stages of drug use: A developmental analysis. *Journal of Youth and Adolescence, 7*, 13–40.

Kandel, D., Simcha-Fagan, O., & Davies, M. (1986). Risk factors for delinquency and illicit drug use from adolescence to young adulthood. *Journal of Drug Issues, 16*, 67–90.

Kelly, J. (1988). A guide to conducting prevention research in the community: First steps. *Prevention in Human Services, 6*(1), whole issue.

Kingery, P. M., Pruitt, B. E., & Hurley, R. S. (1992). Violence and illegal drug use among adolescents: Evidence from the U.S. National Adolescent Student Health Survey. *The International Journal of the Addictions, 27*(12), 1445–1464.

Krosnick, J. A., & Judd, C. M. (1982). Transitions in social influences at adolescence: Who induces cigarette smoking? *Developmental Psychology, 18*, 359–368.

Levine, S. M. (1974). *Narcotics and drug abuse.* Cincinnati, OH: W.H. Anderson Company.

Lorion, R. P., & Ross, J. P. (Eds.) (1992). Programs for change: Office of Substance Abuse Prevention demonstration models [OSAP special issue]. *Journal of Community Psychology*, 3–9.

McKelvy, J. G., Schneider, E., & Johnson, K. W. (1990). *Selection of church communities for the Creating Lasting Connections project: Description of the selection process*, Working Paper No. 3. Louisville, KY: Urban Research Institute and COPES, Inc.

Moskowitz, J.M. (1989). The primary prevention of alcohol problems: A critical review of the research literature. *Journal of Studies on Alcohol, 50*, 54–88.

Musto, D. F. (1987). *The American disease: Origins of narcotic control.* New York: Oxford University Press.

National Institute on Drug Abuse (1997a). *Community readiness for drug abuse prevention: Issues, tips, and tools.* Rockville, MD: Author.

National Institute on Drug Abuse (1997b). *Preventing drug use among children and adolescents.* Rockville, MD: Author.

Nowlis, H. (1975). *Drugs demystified.* Paris: The Unesco Press.

Pransky, J. (1991). *Prevention: The critical need.* Springfield, MO: Burrell Foundation.

Rappaport, J. (1987). Terms of empowerment/exemplars of prevention: Toward a theory for community psychology. *American Journal of Community Psychology, 15*, 121–148.

Reilly, D. (1979). Family factors in the etiology and treatment of youthful drug abuse. *Family Therapy, 11*, 149–171.

Saffer, H. (1991). Alcohol advertising bans and alcohol abuse: An international perspective. *Journal of Health Economics, 10*, 65–79.

Simch-Fagan, O., Gersten, J. C., & Langner, T. (1986). Early precursors and concurrent correlated of illicit drug use in adolescents. *Journal of Drug Issues, 16*, 7–28.

Smith, A. (1975). *Powers of mind.* New York: Random House.

Strader, T., Collins, D., Noe, T., & Johnson, K. (1997). Mobilizing church communities for alcohol and other drug abuse prevention through the use of volunteer church advocate teams. *The Journal of Volunteer Administration, 15*(2), 16–29.

Tec, N. (1974). Parent–child drug abuse: Generational continuity or adolescent deviancy? *Adolescence 9*, 350–364.

Volk, R. J., Edwards, D. W., Lewis, R. A., & Sprenkle, D. H. (1989). Family systems of adolescent substance abusers. *Family Relations, 38*, 266–272.

Wagenaar, A. C. (1993). *Minimum drinking age and alcohol availability to youth: Issues and research needs. Economics and the prevention of alcohol-related problems.* NIAAA Research Monograph 25.

Well, M.O., & Gamble, D.N. (1995). Community practice models. In R. Edwards (Ed.), *Encyclopedia of social work* (19th ed.). Washington, DC: National Association of Social Workers, 577–594.

Werner, E. E. (1989). High-risk children in youth and adulthood: A longitudinal study from birth to 32 years. *American Journal of Orthopsychiatry, 59*, 72–81.

Werner, E. E., & Smith, R. S. (1982). *Vulnerable but invincible.* New York: McGraw–Hill.

Wheelan, S., & McKeage, R. (1993). Developmental patterns in small and large groups. *Small Group Research, 24*, 60–83.

White, W. L. (1979). Themes in chemical prohibition. In *Drugs in perspective, resource manual* (pp. 171–182). Rockville, MD: National Institute on Drug Abuse.

Zander, A. (1994). *Making groups effective* (2nd ed.). San Francisco: Jossey–Bass.

Index